# Praise for *Off the Record*

I am amazed at the dedication required to maintain an effort like this consistently for this length of time. And as it plainly shows, during a time already filled to the brim with activity, events, and a full life. Truly a Pepysian effort!

More than any other writings I have seen, this gives a clear and comprehensive view of the actual experience of Army Nurses in Vietnam, replete with the details like Repl Depot, hootch outfitting, waiting for orders, shortages, memorable patients, coping mechanisms, R&R, ward management, etc. This is a valuable historical resource.

–Colonel Nickey McCasland Ret, US Army Nurse Corps

# "Off The

# RECORD"

7530-222-3524
FEDERAL SUPPLY SERVICE
(GPO)

# Off the Record

**Wisdom Editions**

Minneapolis

First Edition July 2023
*OFF THE RECORD: A Vietnam War Nurse's Journal*
Copyright © 2023 by Felicitus Edith Ferington. All rights reserved.

10 9 8 7 6 5 4 3 2 1

ISBN: 978-1-960250-88-9

Cover and Book design by Gary Lindberg

# Off the Record

A Vietnam War Nurse's Journal

## Fay Ferington

Wisdom
Editions

Minneapolis

# Table of Contents

# Foreword

I served a year with the 1st Infantry Division (Big Red One) in 1967 as a combat medic. I spent my year in the field, pulled countless patrols both day and night, and dealt with everything you can imagine in a war zone. It was my job to render care to soldiers immediately after they were wounded. I did my best and put many injured comrades on a medivac to be taken to an emergency trauma center, where their survival depended on the care they received from our doctors and nurses. If a wounded soldier were alive when I put them on a "dust-off," they had a 92 percent chance of survival. I never knew where the wounded were taken or even if they survived, but I was confident the wounded would be given the best compassionate medical care available anywhere in the world. I was one part of a complex medical treatment system that saved over 300,000 American lives. Those that survived owe a debt of gratitude to the highly skilled nurses who rendered care to the injured under some very difficult situations. These caregiving nurses were destined to a life of remembering the misery of it all.

Colonel Ferington's journal reflects her experiences as a nurse at a field hospital in Vietnam. She expertly writes about trauma, caring for wounded soldiers and praying for those that did not survive their battle injuries. She also discusses the satisfaction garnered by successful treatment and the heartache that all Vietnam veterans experienced when someone died. This journal provides superb insights into the issues of boredom and extreme stress, which were all part of a typical day in a combat zone. These were the things all who served in Vietnam experienced. This journal also takes the reader directly into the line of fire and describes how nurses put broken soldiers back together. Ferington teaches us how combat nurses can creatively overcome adversity and turn it into a positive.

The war in Vietnam taught a generation of Americans about the nastiness of war and the political turmoil that represents the significant divergence of opinions surrounding the morality of decisions made by our politicians. The captivating contents of this journal brings into focus the complex dilemma that faced soldiers and citizens alike. The Vietnam War was about survival, bravery, treating the wounded, despair, and how to deal with the aftermath and madness of it all. Ferington teaches us how to fashion a productive life after experiencing the worst of life as a young adult. Her combat tour of duty prepared her for the challenges she would face in her military career. She not only became a role model as an officer, but she also became a model citizen as well.

The enemy sometimes targeted field hospitals to create chaos and lower the morale of those who were doing their best to save lives. This journal captures those moments and articulates the spirit of positivity necessary to move forward. The author eloquently writes about the guilt, horror, discomfort and indignity we all experienced. She helps us understand what it was like to be terrified but not having time to acknowledge fear until the next day. After all, we had the rest of our lives to deal with remorse and the memories that were imposed by combat treatment. I am thankful that Colonel Ferington shared her story so we can learn from her experiences and fully appreciate how she was able to turn post-traumatic stress into post-traumatic strength.

Bill Strusinski
Author of *Care Under Fire*

# Preface

It's a long way from a small farm in western New York to Vietnam, and I couldn't help but wonder how being there would affect me. When I arrived in Vietnam as an Army nurse on October 22, 1966, one of the first orders we received was that we were not to keep a diary under any circumstances. This surprised me. I had kept a diary during Basic Training. I had wanted a record of what it was like to join the Army, and I sure as heck wanted one of what was going to happen in the coming year of my tour of duty in the war. I had finished nursing school almost six years earlier and since then had obtained a Master of Science degree in psychiatric-mental health nursing. I had never been rebellious, but I decided that I would keep a journal, not a diary. I would only write about my daily activities, and I would show no one.

I looked around Post and found a blank book with the word RECORD stamped on the cover: a blank book intended to keep track of supplies and equipment. In fine print, it read: FEDERAL SUPPLY SYSTEM 7530-222-3524. When a friend wrote "Off the" on the book cover, I had a name for my journal.

*Off the Record* had its beginnings many years prior to my decision to write it. I was four years old when WWII began. The war was a regular part of everyone's life, including the children. Each week on Monday, I gave my teacher, Miss Brown, a dime for the war effort; I picked milkweed pods for parachute silk with my brothers and searched for scrap metal along the railroad tracks. I hid along with the rest of my family during the routine air-raid alerts.

By 1945, at the age of eight, I had learned to read, and was shocked to find out that people killed in the war were known as casualties. I had thought that "casual" meant something not very serious. The next year, I put my feelings into words in the form of a poem called "The Soldier." I really struggled with the last two lines: "Yes in the field where humans lay / he fought in the war that terrible day..."

I was fourteen when my brother, Norm, was sent to fight in Korea. On the farm, it was important that we each carried our part of the workload. Naturally, if Norm was in danger someplace, I needed to help him. I couldn't and felt guilty for a long time afterward.

Ten years later, we all heard the first rumblings of war in Vietnam. I was a student in my master's program at the University of Michigan, where the campus was alive with anti-war protests. I was troubled, but I graduated and soon became heavily committed to my first job as nursing supervisor of the children's program at Ypsilanti State Hospital. The demonstrations grew more radical. By 1966, I could no longer resist getting involved, not in the street activity, but in a deep consideration about my responsibility. Should I help regardless of what the popular view of the war was? They needed nurses. I would be contributing to people's care, in any case. In July of that year, I volunteered for and was commissioned as a captain in the US Army Nurse Corps. I requested and was given a direct assignment to Vietnam.

The decision made, there was little time to think about it. I resigned my position, which by then was director of nursing at the York Woods Center for the care of emotionally disturbed children in Ann Arbor, Michigan. Armed with directions the recruiter sent me, I shopped for a few pieces of clothing and some personal care items that would not be available in a war zone. Number one on my list was a trunk because I was allowed 600 pounds of belongings to be shipped to me shortly after leaving the US. I felt a chill when I explained to the salesperson at Sears that I was going to Southeast Asia.

I packed my household goods and drove them to my parent's home in New York. I didn't know that the Army would have taken care of that for me. I had been to New York City, had once driven to California, and I so was excited about going half a world away to another country in the South China Sea. At times I think I was a little giddy.

One day though, I awoke, and I was afraid. Where and how would I live in Vietnam? Would I be up to whatever demands occurred as a result of the war? How would I adjust? Soon I was there and began to find answers to these questions.

On my first day of duty, my first patient, a twenty-one-year-old Lieutenant with a bandage wrapped about his head, covering his eyes, was arguing with the doctor that he needed to return to the field:

"But you get to go home now," the doctor told him.

"I can't do that. My men need me sir."

The young soldier was blind.

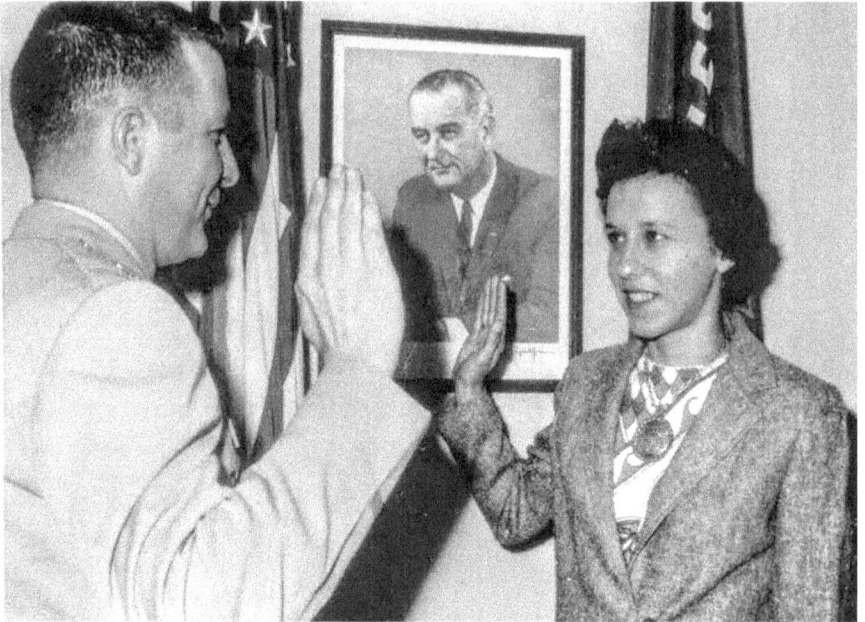

On August 2, 1966, "I swore to defend... against all enemies, foreign and domestic."

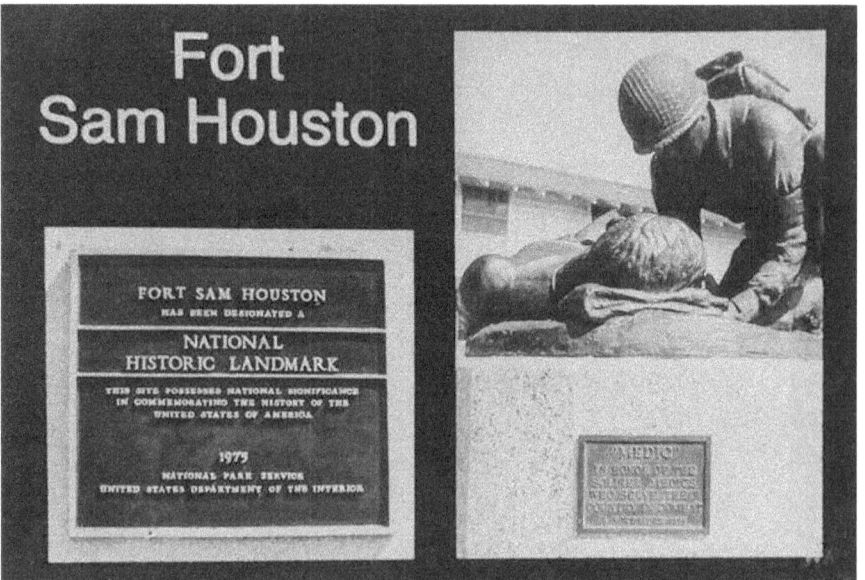

On August 25, 1966, I reported for active duty to "Ft. Sam."

# Chapter 1: Basic Training
# (Early Sep – 26 Oct 1966)

**Early Sep 66**  I don't know the date and haven't had occasion to care. So much has happened since last Monday that I should be keeping a diary. Yesterday, we received our fatigue issue and picked up "cords" from the uniform shop. Tried on the latter after returning from dinner at the Casa Rio. Also, yesterday, we met Col. Parker. He entered and, having been so instructed, we jumped to our feet. I felt a bit conspicuous but needn't have. Everyone moved in full accord. We were divided into platoons and assumed a first formation at the next break (10 AM). Forty-five minutes in 90+ sun. Feet burned right thru the sandals (don't wear uniforms 'til this Mon.); back ached, hand minus its circulation from practicing saluting, arm ached from holding salute, perspiration a small river out of bra and down to skirt band. A couple of kids fainted, and we learned it was their own lack of foresight. One doesn't lock one's knees when assuming attention. Formation again at 2:00 and 3:15, then to publications for book issue and later a class in grade structure. After that, picked up fatigues and field gear. To the Pit (an on-post hang out) at 5:00 for some well-deserved beer.

At the Pit, Shirley looked like she wanted to cry. "I don't know why I join United States Army!" I'm tired, but most happy to be here. I haven't received any letters, though, and that is irritating. I don't feel much like visiting with others tonight. I smile to realize I learned the

# of the girl next to me in formation before I learned her name. The system works, at least temporarily, without our even realizing it. #6 is Nancy. I'm #7 in the 3rd squad. Easy thing to remember,

$$3 \times 7 = 21$$

This must be difficult for kids who not only don't see sense in this sort of thing but can't find stimulation in studying the application of the concept of total institutionalization… for example, last night, in addition to putting on insignia and brass with a ruler… an odd exception, attaching a name plate.

**Today**: Formation at 8:15—breakfast in the consolidated mess—cold toast, tasteless eggs, but the coffee wasn't as bad as rumored. I was musing about whether I'm doing OK or not—must be, only one minor incident to distinguish me from 280 others in "C Company." Wed, after 3 beers, I decide the appearance of our tac officer in the Pit is an occasion for humor and extend a friendly greeting—perhaps too friendly. Later I heard that he felt so little pain, he fell right out of his chair. No worry there, I guess.

I've become irate with the system only once Thursday, taking an aptitude test. Being in the aisle seat position, I received tests for the whole row and, through habit, turned them face down. The Major immediately and without comment took the exams and turned them back face up. It wouldn't do to inform that man that I had reason for my behavior. He didn't ask anyway.

The first week was long and hard for some of the kids. Actually, it's not nearly as bad as I had feared it might be. I might even make it. Last Monday, however, everybody was bubbly and talkative for about 6 hours. By 5 PM today, there wasn't one smiling face (including the men). Maybe these few days were designed to impress upon us who is "boss." They did indeed run the hell out of us.

Some moments have been frustrating… spruce up for the ID picture, and it comes out looking like…? Get fitted for dress blues and then have to put the cords back on. Granny shoes are purchased, and I do believe Major Mahoney's statement, "They will be your best friends for the next 6 weeks." My feet hurt and swell considerably. They try hard to be firm with us (ex: "If the car of a general officer passes and it appears empty, salute. If you wish, you can assume the general is on the floor and that's why he's not visible") but a fellowship keeps intruding, and we wind up at a happy medium. However, what with the pace of the schedule, the heat and the strangeness of each day's experiences, the group isn't too amenable to cheering, so I say little about anticipating working at real nursing in RVN (Republic of Vietnam) and either gripe right along or remain quiet. Besides, to do otherwise might exceed the energy/fatigue ratio.

**19 Sep 66** Been studying several hours for an exam in Military Science. Have discovered the last couple of days that keeping well-groomed in uniform is nearly a full-time job... washed uniforms earlier—still must iron them, put on brass (polish it first) and polish shoes. Became keyed up yesterday thinking it would be necessary to lead the 1st Platoon in drill, as was the case Friday noon. Fortunately (or not), the rain broke just after report, and we double-timed it to class. The door to the building was locked, and it was necessary to reroute to the next area. We were drenched.

At least it was cooler this weekend. Last Thursday was nearly brutal, with over 5 hours of continuous class after a 1030 lunch break. These past 2 weeks have gone rapidly, and much continues to be new. Most of us average between 3 to 6 hours of sleep nightly. For the most part, we could manage 8 hours, but that would allow no time for complaints and speculations regarding PCSs (permanent change of station).

Summary:

1) Gen. Collin's reception

2) class on how to do trachs (trachiotomy) and infusions

3) morale of the first platoon is admirable

**20 Sep 66**   Listed the above topics as they occurred in the past 2 weeks but was too tired to elaborate. Today was a good one, even tho' I had only 2 hours of sleep the second night in a row. My window looks directly east, and having arisen at sunrise, the lights of the heart of San Antonio shown clearly, and the sky was a deep pink. The post flag stood in silhouette.

Monday (last night) I noticed the uniform could stand improvement. Apparently, one uses toothpaste on one's brass. It took 2 hours to "spit-shine" the shoes, but I emerged triumphant (and with muscle strain in the shoulders—oh my sedentary past)! How narcissistic they must wish us to be. Everything should be in fine shape for the in-ranks inspection this Friday. Everyone will be in dress blues except those with a direct assignment to RVN. I will be proud to wear greens—vanity I'm afraid.

**22 Sep 66**   Tomorrow we begin an orientation to Vietnam. I am eager to get on with some important activity. The number of girls who have volunteered for an assignment there is interesting. One has a fiancé at Qui Nhon, and she will leave after an interim assignment at William Beaumont in El Paso. Most have no such "legitimate" reason, including myself. Someone kiddingly proposed a reunion of C and A companies for Christmas in RVN.

Today was mentioned as "being good." Dawn was followed by an extra-special breakfast; in formation by 0710. By then, the sun was bright and warm (not hot and wet as is the case about noon). A breeze blew, the quad was filled (including a company of Medical Service Corps Officers who are newer than we are), and the band was present. The kids looked sharp and later were most enthusiastic regarding the band. They played the Army Nurse Corps song, and I thought, "what a nice march" without realizing until halfway through what it was.

Class was fairly interesting. Also, we had our first long break since we arrived. I have been asked to speak at Company C's graduation (Dress Blue Dinner for all 280 of us), and I accepted. Mail was the event of the day. I received my Port-of-Call (port for departing CONUS, i.e., Continental United States): Travis Air Force Base on October 20th... one month from today. I read and reread the P of C. It seems hard to believe. It is strange to link that with the information we received about techniques of "special warfare."

Announcements: 1) Yes, we will go to Camp Bullis for the field exercise (good!); 2) there will be no in-quarters inspection on the 27th; and 3) more aptitude testing tomorrow at 6:15 (whoops, 1815). Captains who are not platoon leaders are excused, and with everyone so occupied, it should be a good time to study.

I have met some very good people here, and that helps, but last night was bad in terms of feelings of isolation. So rarely does anyone allow feelings and thoughts to appear through the patter and gripes that it is becoming tiresome.

**0100 on 02 Oct 66**   Just finished packing for Camp Bullis. Radio is playing "Cherish," pistol belt all set with poncho, canteen, first-aid pack... duffle bag is full. Ready for the field! Ginny cut my hair tonight and set it; a little differently than I would have... maybe a new way to wear it though it won't make much difference starting on 22 Oct. We'll wear baseball caps in RVN, and that will take care of any style. Several weeks have passed rapidly. We will be essentially finished at Ft. Sam this week, with Bullis and the last exam behind us. Just one more week. It will be hard to leave so many new friends.

I have been happy here, and regardless of what happens, this, at least, has been experienced. Will I really get to RVN and contribute in what will become a "routine"? That is not to imply a series of dull events, but rather, could the implications of my orders ever reach the point of being an expected aspect of one's daily life? Will there be someone there to keep distance and hard work from becoming a burden? Mary Jo is going to Alabama, Ginny to Walter Reed, Jan to Denver as well as Phyllis.

**04 Oct 66** This AM (0500) life, it really seems like we're in the Army. I've been up since 0230, having had "fire-watch" from 0300 to 0400. It was hot in the tent, and I was so disorganized that it finally appeared best to give up on sleeping. I took my duffle bag to the latrine, where it was emptied and repacked. After a leisurely public shower, I dressed in damp fatigues. The mess tent (hall?) consists of rows of tables just tall enough to lean on. That saves space that otherwise would have been used for benches upon which one might have sat. It's still dark... one good note, there was hot coffee and ice water available at 0430. I must say that it seemed like the night couldn't have been worse.

1500 and we are awaiting a demonstration of air-evac techniques... just talking with Mary Jo regarding the difficulty of giving people a real picture of what we do each day. We are about the grubbiest 280 people around. It was very hot today. We had only 15 minutes for lunch, which didn't sit well with me. We then went to a class on the use of the gas mask and a weapons demonstration, followed by a lecture and a physical exercise on the use of the field radio and phone.

**06 Oct 66** Back at Ft. Sam. The more pictures taken, the less the inclination to write. Everyone appears aware of the inevitability of separating. I'm a photo bug almost anytime, but it seems that everyone has been bitten recently. (Maybe it can be retained if it is recorded often enough.) Bullis wasn't so bad. We can put on a gas mask in less than 9 seconds, know how to shoot a 45, and saw how devastating a 57-mm rifle can be at 800 meters. We can use a mess kit without spilling breakfast, can "form up" in the dark, go to the latrine and shower in each other's company, set up a field hospital, use a C-ration can opener and roll a poncho even during classes.

Today was my birthday and was celebrated with dinner and dancing at the Pit. It was a heartwarming gesture on the part of Mary Jo and Ginny. Had a test in Nursing Science; the last one... good to finish that. We turned in the field gear and got malaria pills and some additional immunizations. We leave here next Friday.

**15 Oct 66** Yesterday, we completed the 7-week basic orientation at Ft. Sam, packed, said goodbyes and made it precisely 123 miles toward El Paso... stopping at Junction City. It's noon. The weather is cool and the terrain scenic. The road is two-lane, gradually climbing, lots of curves but little traffic. The experience at Ft. Sam was so intense, but today it has proven elusive. Was graduation only slightly over 24 hours ago, and did I say goodbye to Ginny, Ed, Mary Jo, Dick, Linda, Fred, and Joanne only then? Ginny said, "We'll all be with you." At first, I thought she meant by way of thoughts and letters (as I will be with them), but perhaps she meant it literally.

Graduation was surprisingly pleasant, though undeniably tinged with nostalgia. This was that of which people spoke in high school and college and which was so faintly present then. I have eaten, worked, worried, played, laughed, and griped with you as we shared all kinds of lectures, exams, and films about RVN. Which of us will be touched as these things become reality? Six weeks ago, the Army Nurse Corps song was sung faintly out of self-consciousness (or perhaps a mild distaste for some of the words). Today it was sung faintly out of emotion. God go with you, my friends...

**17 Oct 66** Henderson, Nevada: I don't understand clearly the reasons for volunteering for Vietnam... perhaps a fling at adventure, a flair for the dramatic, but more certainly than any reason is a need to give (not more), but more keenly than is required in most day-to-day circumstances. I think my character fit for what I shall encounter.

How fortunate is one to have traversed the country prior to such an encounter, who has intimate recall of the object of his work. My pity to those who have now or will yet give their life without having known our country... without knowing that the hills are soft and green in Vermont and Massachusetts and New York, without having known that the forests of Northern Michigan are lush in their virginity, or that wheat in Kansas is nearly red when ripe. My pity to that person who has not seen the arid mountains of Nevada, the magnificence of a Texas sky, the white sand of the Gulf of Mexico, or known the utter stillness of the valleys across the bay from San Francisco.

## *En Route:*

**21 Oct 66**   By California time, it's 7:35 PM, which means it's 4:30 AM in Anchorage, where we stopped briefly but didn't get off the plane. In view of the fact that we can't be more than an hour away from Japan, neither of these times is applicable. I do believe it's still Friday here in the plane though it's approaching Saturday AM in Japan. It will take several more hours to get from Japan to Saigon. We'll get there mid-Saturday AM. (Announcement on the intercom just now: 25 minutes out of Japan at 11:30 PM their time.) This would make a crazy schedule to punch a clock by…

The pilot started his descent. We'll be here on the ground for 2 hours. The AFB (Air Force Base) Yakota, is large, drab and rather restricted. "No photos, stay in the roped-off area, etc." (It's 8:45 AM San Francisco time.) Coming in over Tokyo, there were blocks of lights as far as one could see. The night was remarkably clear. We left Travis AFB 14.5 hours ago, and it is still dark.

Connie, Barb, Donna and Charlotte saw us off at Travis AFB. Us refers to Cathy, Loren, myself and Tony. We met the guys the night before at a club. While dancing, Loren told me he was leaving for RVN the next day. I said, "I am too!" He must have been surprised, for my white off-the-shoulder dress gave no hint. As it turns out, we were scheduled for the same flight.

I forgot to mention one minor item: Flight 243 is compliments of Pan Am. Cathy the stewardesses and myself are the only women in a group of about 200 people. It's 3:30 AM Saturday, Tokyo time. In San Francisco, it's around noon, but it's Friday.

We had an additional 1½ hours at that last stop to repair a water leak. Just took off, the last leg of the flight—about 6½ hours to go.

We've had three different crews, would you believe? You should see how these greens are holding up. They don't even look like they've been slept in. I wish the feet could be elevated. It would encourage venous return, thereby increasing the size of everyone's shoes.

Cathy and Tony are sleeping. Loren's in the latrine. We are about to be served coffee, but upon reaching for the sweet rolls we had stashed under the window, we found that they had been cleaned out along with the ashtrays. Hence, I will skip the coffee. Live and learn about travel...

"Good morning, men." (The captain obviously didn't scan his passenger roster before taking off.) "We're cruising at about 28,000 feet. Sorry for the delay in Yakota. We hope to offer a pleasant trip from here in. The weather... etc., etc. It's 62 degrees in Saigon." I miscalculated the time to go yet. Everybody (not everybody, an overuse of superlatives again) has his or her watch on a different time. Loren suggested we consolidate and call it "infantry-nurse corps time."

How about 20 hours down and 4 to go. It's 4 AM in Saigon, Saturday. Here the sky appears to be struggling with a sunrise, and we're having a turkey dinner. The sunrise will be the first one since Thursday AM, and it'll be Saturday when we land.

We were talking earlier about where these people will go and briefly what awaits them. One often doesn't speak of what is generally shared in thought. Perhaps one shouldn't. How undramatic drama really is. One-half hour to the airport, according to a stewardess. Daylight has finally arrived, and the turkey breakfast wasn't bad after all.

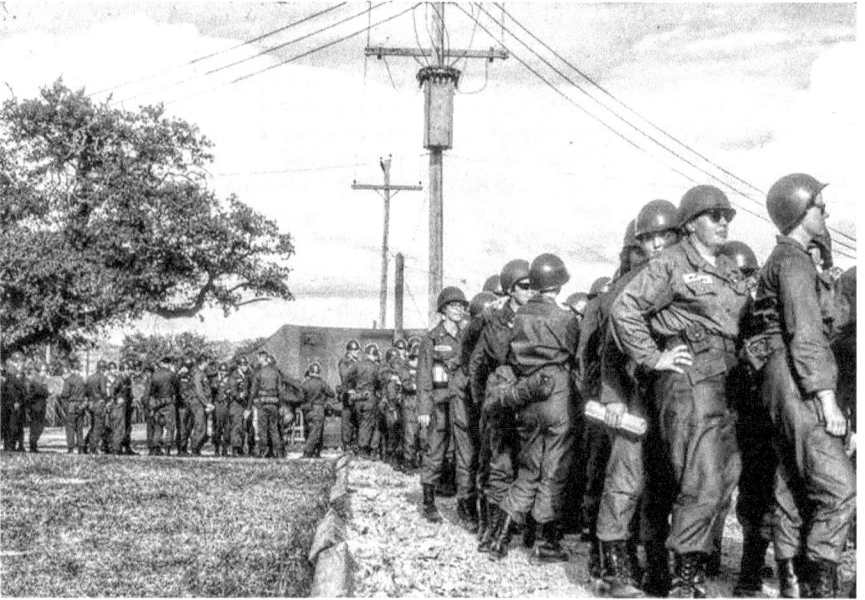

**At Camp Bullis. This is the name of the camp.**

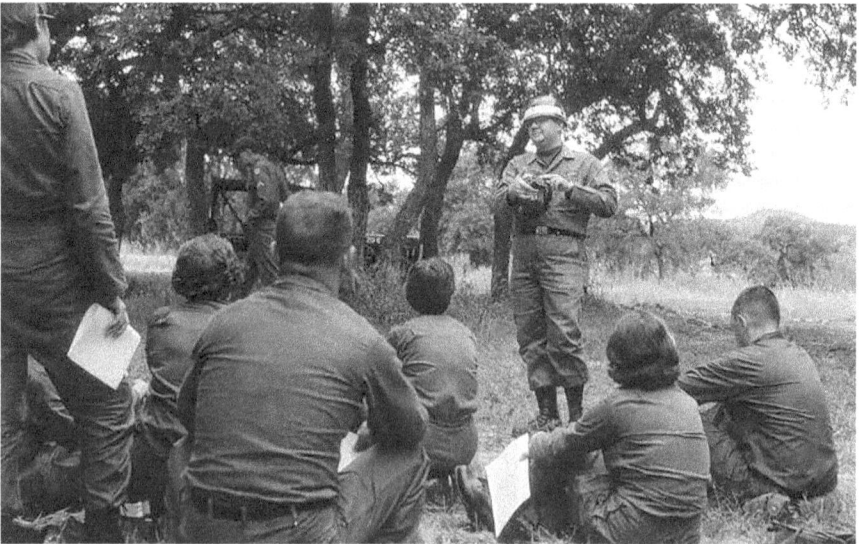

Class

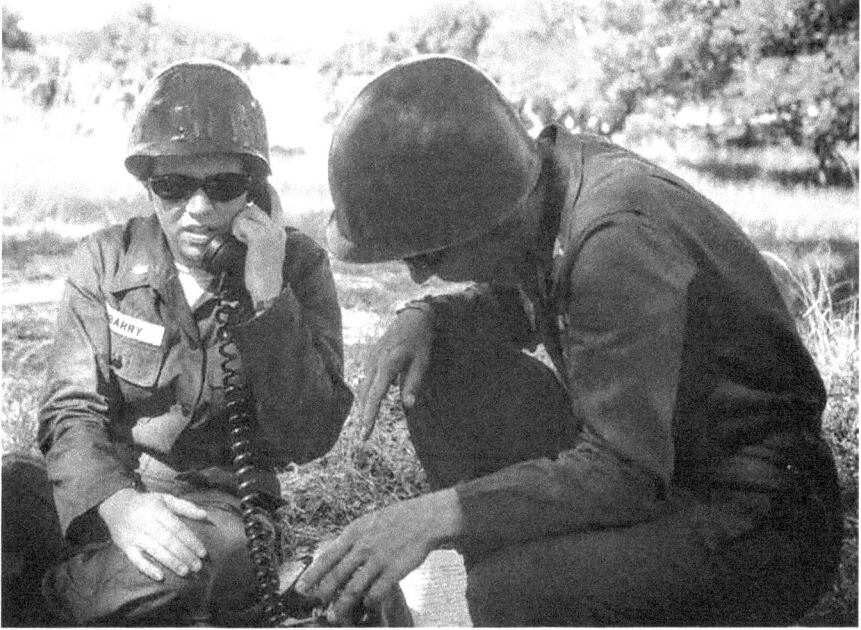

**Use of Field Phone and Radio**

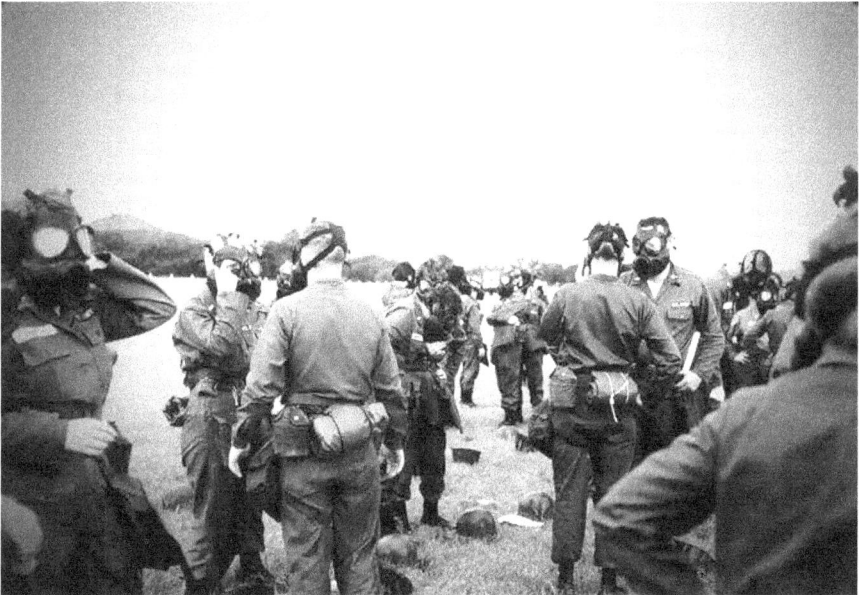

**Gas Chamber Drill**

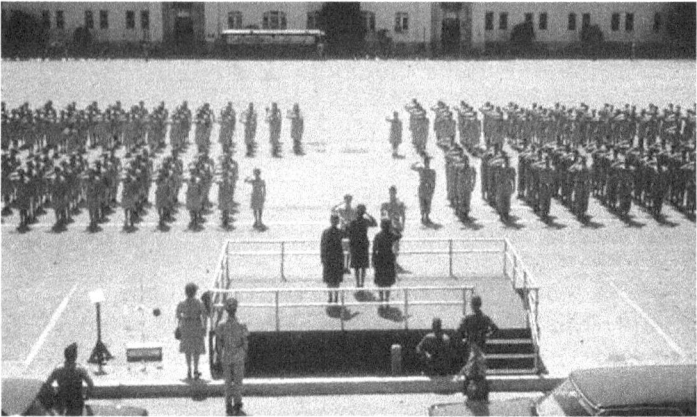

Graduation

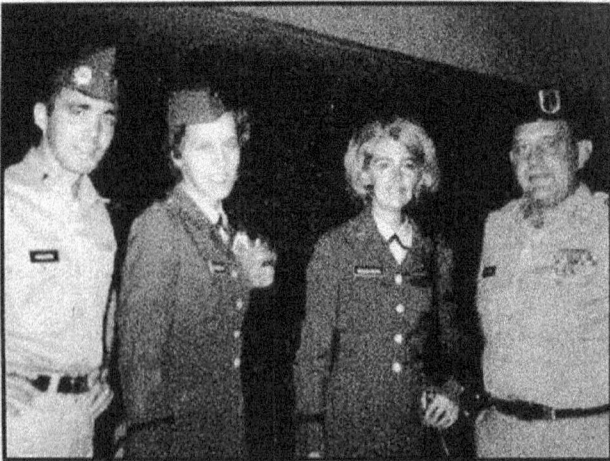

This orchid is the spirit of
"company C" going with
you to nam nam. God
Bless and take care of
our captain ____

Lieutenants {
    Bix
    Donnah
    wear
    Connie
}

Travis Airforce Base

# Chapter 2: In Country
## (28 Oct – 01 Dec 1966)

**28 Oct 66: (one week later)**  I'm sitting on the ward after a very large explosion. It might have been an atomic bomb for all we knew. It was the ammunitions dump instead. We'd heard there was one around here someplace.

Explanation: Colonel C. told us to go to "duty stations" just after the thing went off. I grabbed some cigarettes and my "pot" (helmet) before coming up here. Most of the GIs (patients) were pretty disturbed. Ken "hit the dirt" along with the others, though he'd been having severe shoulder pain all afternoon. It took about 45 minutes to help him realize that nothing had hit him, that he was in the hospital, not the field. He kept calling for a friend who he thought had been hit also. He was the only one of the guys who didn't snap out of it right away.

The building we had been in, near the BOQ (bachelor officers' quarters), was blown 6 inches off its foundation. I wonder where Tony and the other guys went after we left there. It's not safe to do any traveling at this hour. The all clear sounded. Funny, it took people much less time to react tonight than during last night's practice alert.

**30 Oct 66** Two more satchel charges were found in the ammo dump, and the place is alive with rumors. There were 11 casualties from last night's attack, including 2 GI KIAs (killed in action).

**14 Nov 66**  Having written everyone (and the brother thereof), I have the luxury of writing simply to clarify feelings and/or thoughts… one problem, sometimes the letters have served to greatly dilute the awareness of given responses. It's 2300 and "lights out" (we live in a large Quonset hut, with open bay accommodations) except having constructed a type of "hooch" with the aid of a locally acquired straw mat, I am able to turn on the tensor and continue writing.

Today went well. Work is becoming more adequately organized, and having received 2 letters, one from Ginny—one from mother—I found increased energy to devote not just to the GIs but to the staff as well. Tonight, dinner was actually quite good; later I washed, polished the boots to an adequate sheen (something done only by non-combatants) and watched the evening movie. The film "And Now Miguel" was tender and beautiful, portraying the strivings of a lad on the verge of manhood. So many scenes in the movie were made all the more poignant because they paralleled the reality in which I now found myself—the muffled sounds of small arms fire accompanied by the thumping of outgoing artillery, "that lad" being admitted to the 93$^{rd}$, yesterday, today and tomorrow and a med evac chopper leaving a nearby landing pad.

**16 Nov 66**  Tonight already, and yet such a long day. We were at a near standstill on the ward. On Medcap (medical program) afterward, there was only a small group of Vietnamese. Medcap is part of the civil action portion of the war. Medical personnel set up clinics in neighboring villages and provide care to whoever shows up. Sometimes it's a huge event. The evening passed quietly until 2030 when an alert was called.

We went to the bunker, only to discover that it was a false alarm. Pat made a pot of coffee, and a few of us broke bread together… VN bread at that… bread and marmalade and coffee… sheer elegance for a change. We spoke of the alert, of friendship, of the cat and mouse game that surrounds us here. We are X number of people with X amount of defense. We are responsible for 100 to 200 or 300 patients, and at times a feeling of vulnerability is unavoidable. For example:

last evening, we were to get together with the chopper pilots at their club. Today rumor is that a grenade was tossed through the window there, causing extensive damage. Our readiness to believe that rumor without checking it out is the vulnerability of which I speak. There's so much talk of the 93$^{rd}$ being mortared that I've nearly come to regard such as inevitable. Perhaps in one year, I will look back and smile and regard the "reality" of it with raised brow. Tonight, I wonder if I'll ever see the US again. Tonight, another alert.

Reporting for duty, my hand shook as I signed in. A curiosity about the "hour" we were to wait for anticipated VC "activity" induced a giddy tension in patients and staff alike. I wondered if I would maintain the necessary overt calm. I thought foolishly of a film I had once seen (in AZ; Aug 66) and, as did the nurse therein, applied lipstick and combed my hair. I reread the alert procedure, making notifications as required, observing that patients confined to bed would have to be covered… and then the announcement that the alert had been called off and the release of bitching about the inefficiency of any information we get… the self-conscious expression of gratitude for the closeness of friendship. Tonight, we'll sleep but with our clothes and "pot" where they can be accessed in a hurry if need be.

**20 Nov 66**  How vast had been my world these few weeks, and now it's simply a routine of: work, freshen up, write letters, eat dinner, hang around listening to music, check out the nightly movie and make preparations for the next AM of work. Often, emotion crowds out words with another human being; how meaningful are previously unthought-of sounds and sights and odors.

A letter to Ginny:

We often just sit and wait. Sometimes it seems unreal. For the most part, we are very safe; however, should something happen, I have chosen to be here, am participating gratefully in such service, and am convinced that one can rarely live (in the most meaningful sense) without occasionally entertaining a risk to one's personal welfare. Of course, I wish to live but think I would, at the same time, have no compunctions about dying for the United States.

Realizing these things, I further realize that my comments tonight are neither morbid nor dramatic. They are facts with which everyone lives. With these reassurances, loved ones need not worry but simply join one another in a fervent prayer for the day when we will meet again or for the strength to accept never meeting again should such be the outcome of the course of events.

**22 Nov 66 Digression** Four weeks ago yesterday, we arrived in Vietnam. The countryside was quite lovely from above and quite inelegant from the ground. From where the plane stopped, we proceeded to the airport itself (Tan Son Nhut); it was 0900, and it started to rain. We were addressed collectively and initial in country processing began. The terminal was an omen of what was to come; a somewhat garish exterior and a crude, ill-contrived and dirty interior (complete with non-potable water and Vietnamese who were ("not allowed to carry our baggage")… a lot of paperwork and milling around. Afterward, we waited for a ride while our driver was liberally chewed out for not having checked his vehicle for booby-traps. We headed then toward what turned out to be the nearby town of Bien Hoa.

We bumped through the compound to a main street and continued to bump along on a highway of reddish mud. The rain did not let up. There was a lot of traffic as small European taxis darted in and out of a conglomeration of military personnel carriers, construction equipment, motor scooters, bicycles, and pedestrians. Apparently, a miss of 6 inches was considered as good as a miss of three feet with respect to collisions. Had we not previously become somewhat accustomed to the prospect of personal risk, we would have at that time. I thought to myself that, in a sense, the highways were a metaphor for the violence known intimately in the neighboring jungle. Life is somewhat expendable in either place.

Miles through town to Highway 1 afforded a panoramic view of poverty, of skinny barefooted kids, of slight adult figures bent with the labor at hand, of open markets (including slabs of meat) placed casually next to fly-infested mounds of refuse, of roles of barbed wire surrounding an occasional villa, of unsmiling faces under round straw hats… and of an azure billboard with the bold message: Fly Pan AM… eventually the rain subsided.

Surprise #1: Highway 1 rather closely resembles our expressways… though without the median. Bridges are carefully constructed and carefully guarded. Traffic moved more rapidly as it was thinned of scooters and bicycles, which were replaced by additional military vehicles. We drove past rectangles of mud (rice paddies?) through which people moved. An occasional water buffalo waded slowly before its owner. Approximately 20 miles out, our driver embarked on phase 2 of the trip, a trial-and-error approach to the 90th Replacement Center. "No, we're not the replacements for your laundry workers." And in response, "We process only enlisted people here." Finally, we arrived at the location where we were to be registered as newly arrived nurses.

We spent the weekend at the replacement center, where we experienced surprise #2, #3, etc. The CO (Commanding Officer) of the place (Col. Howard) had contacted the 93rd requesting permission for us to report for duty on Monday AM rather than that afternoon. It seems that one of the few buildings among the array of tents and huts was a recently completed officer's club. We (Mac and I) and 4 or 5 other nurses spent Saturday evening in a sandbagged, air-conditioned room listening to a Filipino band play the US Hit Parade and dancing. The music was enhanced as champagne was uncorked, and the party ended with an all-night singalong (which I accompanied with my guitar). While frolicking, we learned that a home is called hooch, the red mud is called laterite, and it's easy to fall asleep after 36 hours of such an assailment of the senses.

**24 Nov 66 Thanksgiving**  It was Thanksgiving… and this was so in every location throughout the Republic of Vietnam, be that "location" a Quonset hut, a tent or an ill-defined area of jungle covered only by strips of startling blue sky. At any rate, today's sunrise was the most unusual of any since we arrived here. In the relative chill of morning, it was almost possible to imagine a Vietnamese Spring.

For us, lunch was turkey and fruit and nutmeats spilled in careful array on a table in the center of the mess hall. There was the light chatter or occasional laugh of the mama-sans as they dished out the food. For those in the field, there were hot meals flown in by chopper, but only if they were not being shot at at the time or if they weren't patrolling in a rice paddy or napping in a hole that they'd just had to dig. Some comparison. We have it so good, and still feel free to complain.

**28 Nov 66**  This commentary is getting a little on the heavy side. Today I was off, and having grown tired of having to move a chair every time I wished to open the dresser drawer and then move it back in order to open the wall locker, I set out in search of a locally made bookcase. It will provide shelves for odds and ends and yet take up less room than a bedside stand. My area is 5' 10" square, but there's 34" of space by the bed. That's where the bookcase will go.

Some hours later… no bookcase. There were dressers and cabinets and chairs and beds, but nothing that even vaguely resembled a bookcase. In the meantime, I took pictures. I tried to counteract the "halo" effect of color film. Viet Nam has unusually impressive skies, and the foliage records as a deep green; hence, it's difficult to capture the shoddy misery of this country.

To summarize, the chairs were covered with worn plastic and the wooden furniture was poorly finished with drawers that opened or closed with considerable difficulty; there were beer-can-backed mirrors with frames of rusting tin and water basins that bent with the pressure of carrying them filled with water. I grew wary at the sight of

GI insecticides and C-rations sold openly at the local market. At one point, I bought a loaf of French bread carefully wrapped in a newspaper from Indiana. Lastly, there were signs all around: "Saigon Ice," "GI come here" and "Car Wash," where children washed vehicles while the GI drivers sought comfort inside from the mothers.

**29 Nov 66**  Just a comment on the weekend that followed. To say the least, it was unexpected. One of the Generals was leaving for home, and his replacement decided to throw a party for the occasion. He sent his helicopter to the 93rd. He wanted the company of some nurses. The Chief Nurse was apparently required to oblige. I volunteered to go.

At the Division Base Camp, the highlight of the evening was an elegant dinner, complete with flowers and candles. There were white table clothes, and there was wine. It was unbelievable. We stayed overnight. We had to sleep in a trailer, though, and with the heat and the mosquitos, we were miserable. An armed GI spent the night outside our door.

The next day (Sunday), we took the General's chopper to Tay Ninh, near the Cambodian border, to visit the 45th Surg. The ground over which we flew was heavily pockmarked with various-sized craters. There were occasional villages that had been leveled, presumably by the recent Operation Attleboro. We flew near a bombing and actually saw the missiles fall from the plane. The smoke below was heavy. I snapped photos of this area of fury. Is one to be awed by such an experience or horror-stricken by the violence? In reality, I was neither…

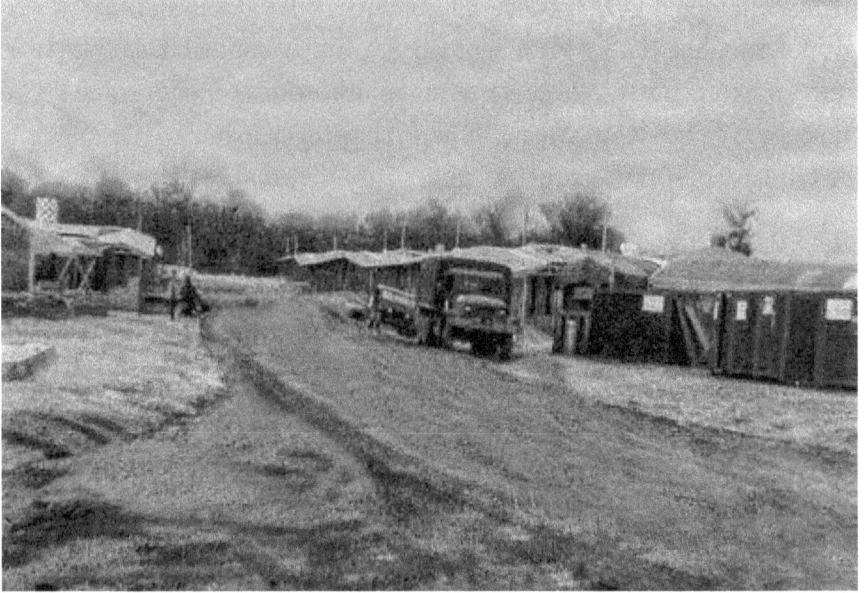

**First Day at 93rd Evacuation Hospital**

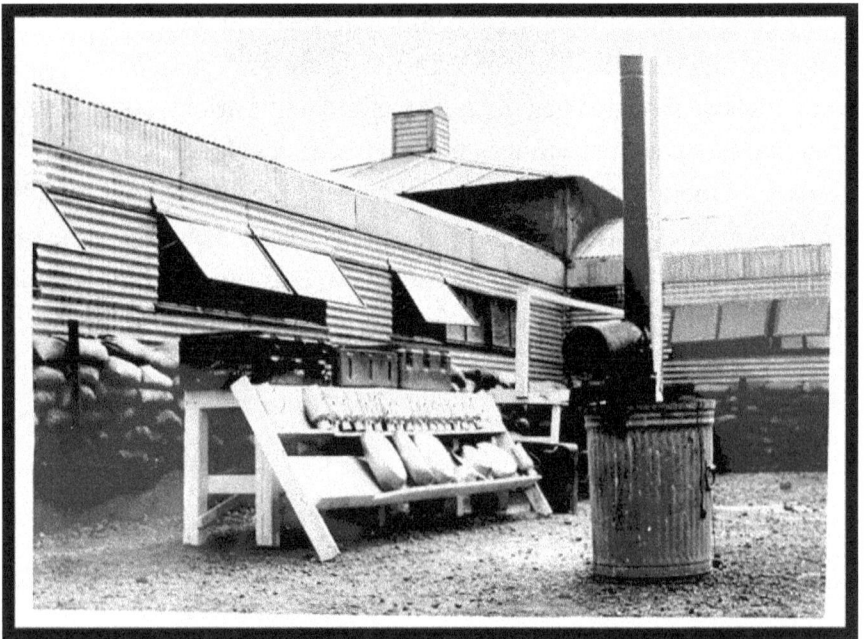

**My clinical unit Ward 4**

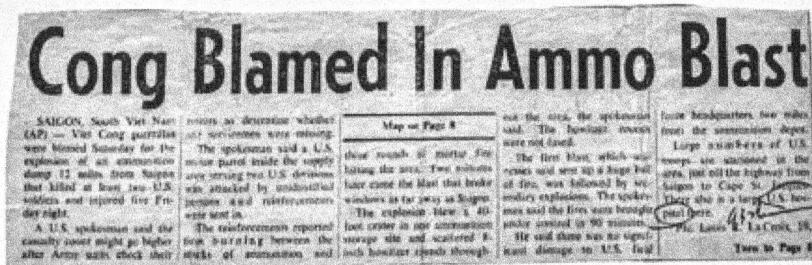

Coverage from the United States

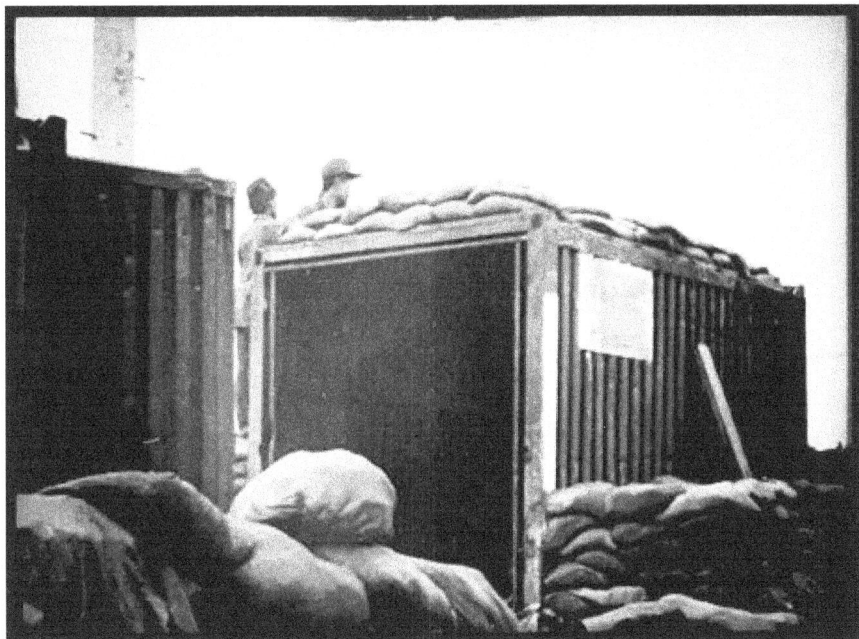

Shipping Crate, Bunker and/or Prison Cell

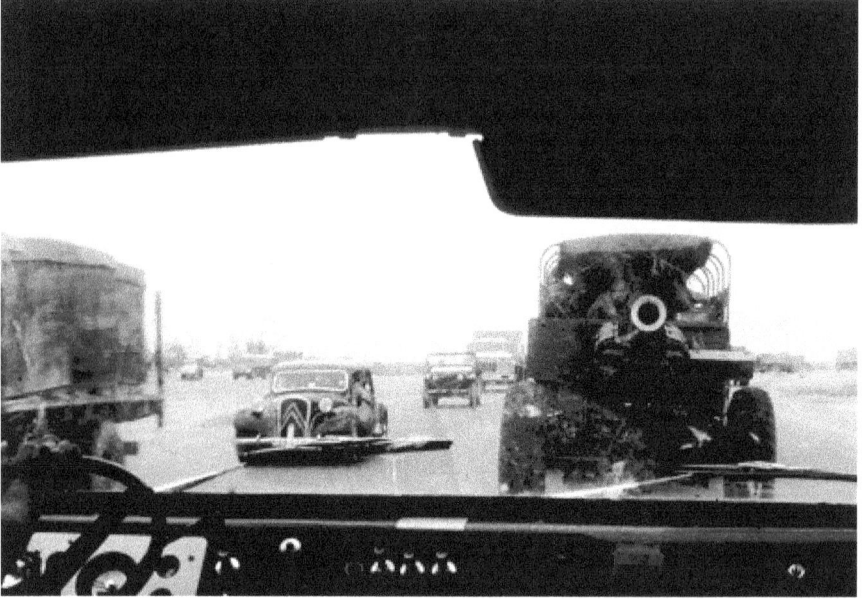

**En Route to Replacement Center**

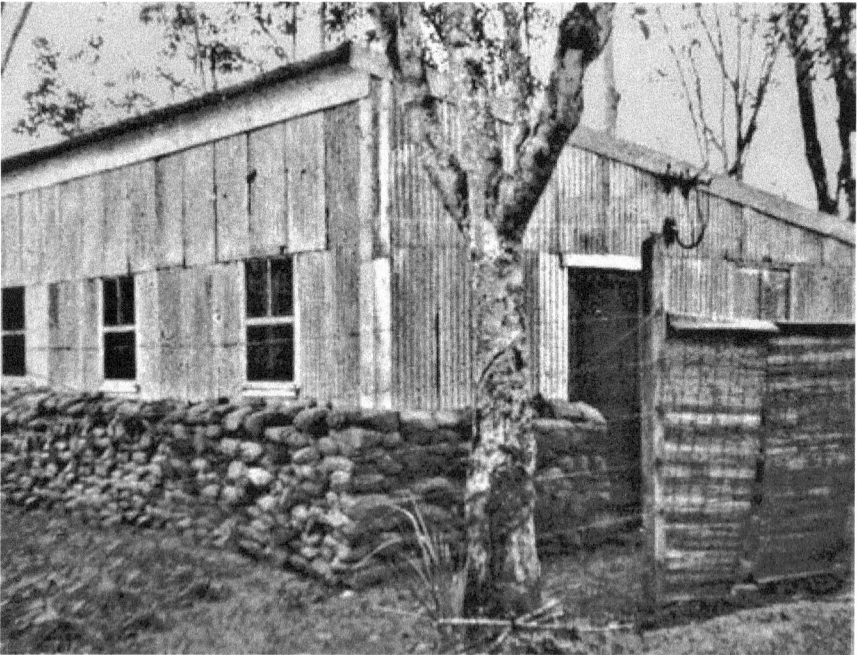

**Nurses' BOQ at 90th Replacement Center**

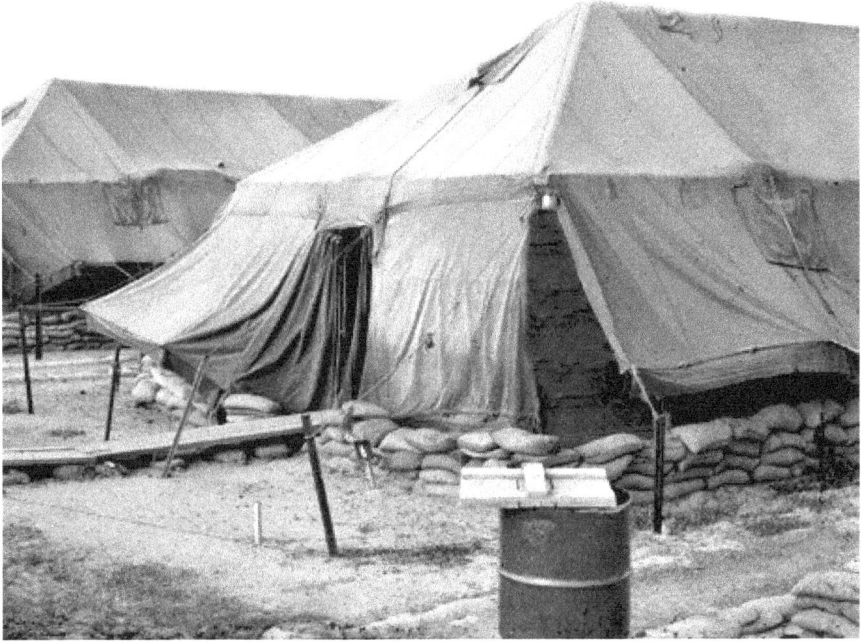

Most Troops Still In Tents At the 90th

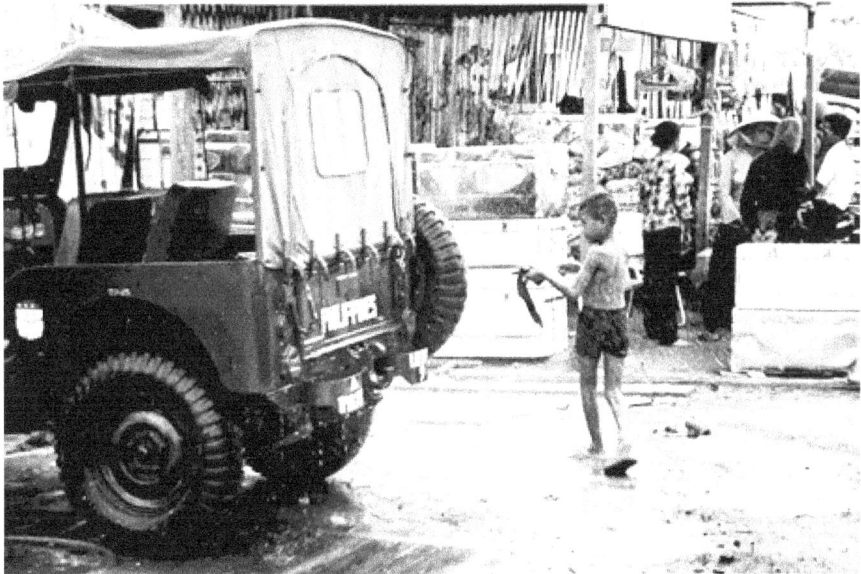

Car Wash

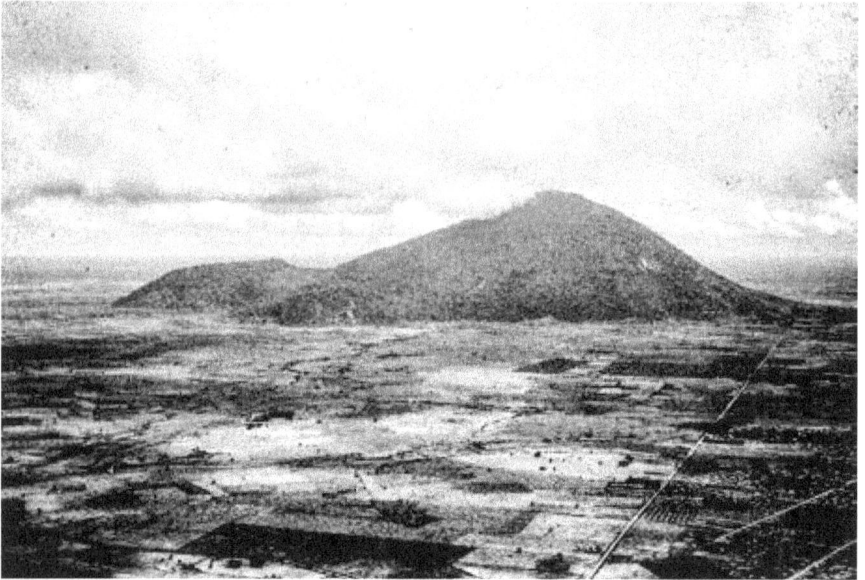

The Black Lady (Tay Nhin), Near Cambodia

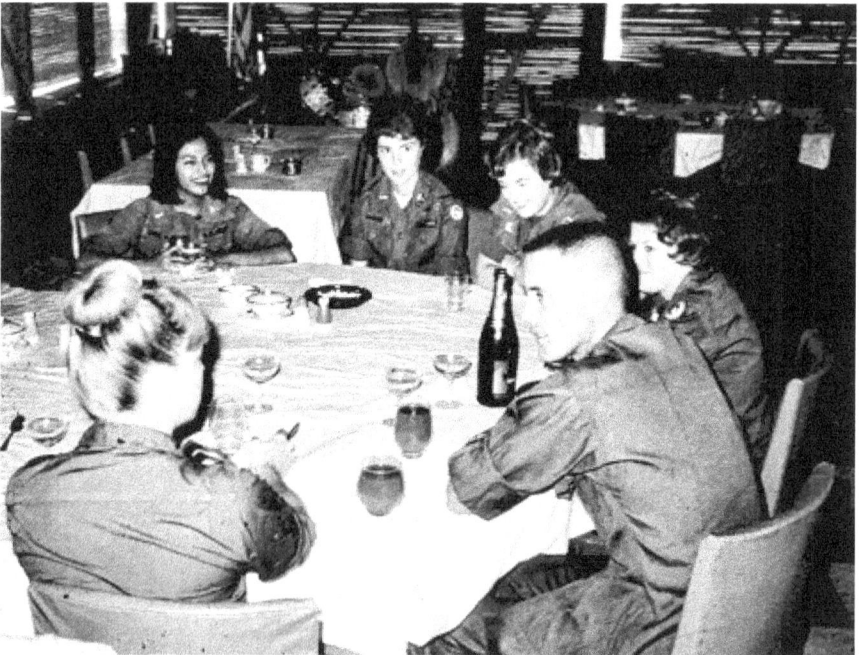

The General's Party (173rd Base Camp)

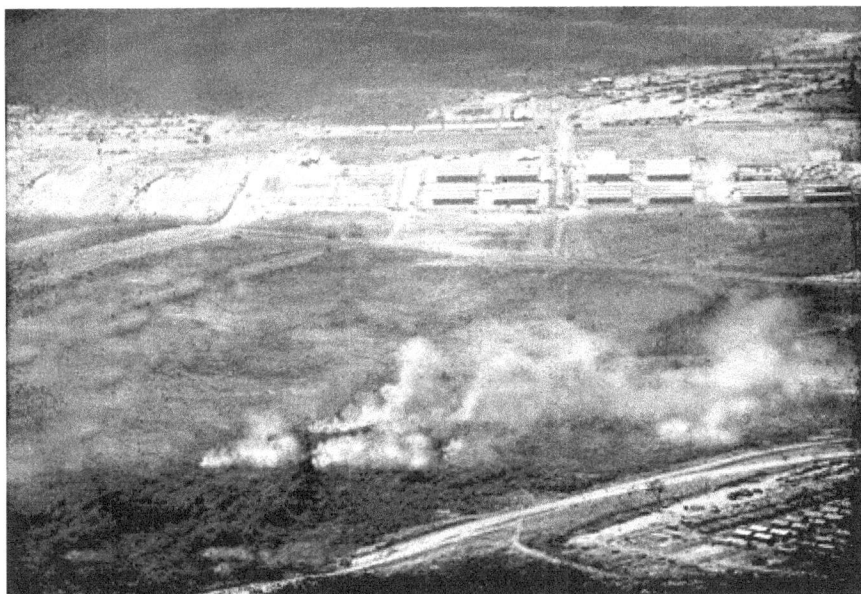

Nearby Activity

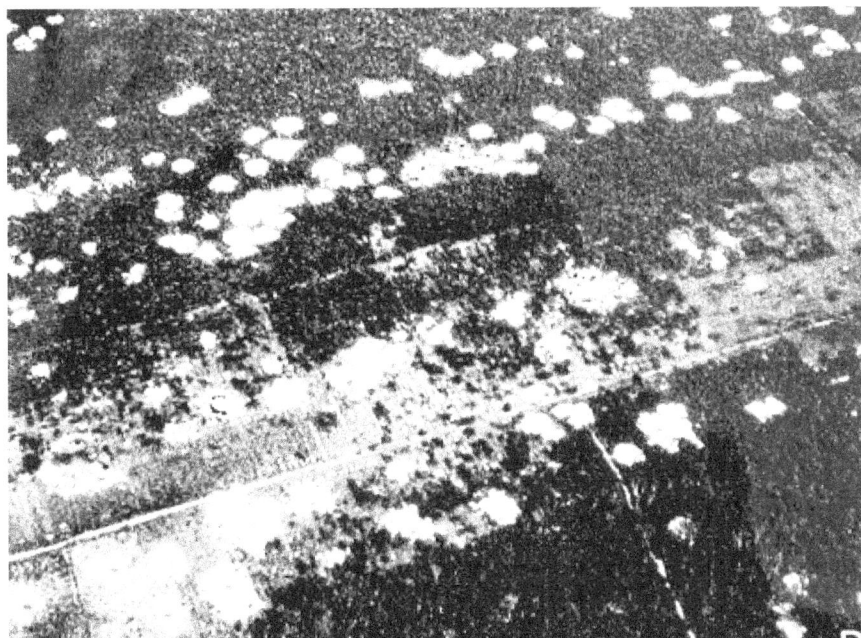

Bomb Craters

# VC Charge Found at Blast Site

S&S Vietnam Bureau

SAIGON — Explosive Ordnance Disposal men found a second satchel charge Saturday morning following an attack on the U.S. Army ammunition depot at Long Binh Friday night.

The EOD men found the charge tied to a pole near a stack of 105mm artillery shells. A military spokesman said the charge had a wristwatch timer attached which had stopped with 50 minutes to go before detonation.

The depot was rocked by a satchel charge Friday evening when a stack of 8-inch unfused howitzer projectiles were blown. The explosion, which could be seen in Saigon, 13 miles away, hurled fragments throughout the area and caused several secondary explosions.

The blast blew a crater about 150 feet by 100 feet and nearly 20 feet deep.

The attack on the depot began when a security patrol came under fire from both automatic weapons and grenades. A few minutes later, the first of three mortar rounds was reported. A U.S. spokesman said that U.S. casualties were light as was material damage to the depot.

News article (Two GIs were killed)

# Chapter 3: A Newbie
# (02 Dec 66 – 02 Jan 67)

**02 Dec 66**   I'm just lying here thinking about one of the last nights in the States. Barb and I had stopped in Las Vegas en route to Travis and spent an evening at the Sands Hotel. We had dinner and later were entranced listening to Lena Horne. The microphone didn't appear to be between her and her audience. Strange that one can be so eager to be done with luxury. Methinks it's rather like too much strawberry shortcake. How good it tastes when one has had none for a while and how tiresome it becomes when the garden is overflowing, as it was that night.

An even 100 degrees in the shade today, but it didn't even seem that warm except around noon. Work went well, and this afternoon we went out on Medcap (to win the hearts and minds). This time it was more interesting—a hundred people or more each with his ache or pain. Some of the children were pathetically neglected. No tears today; progress, I wonder. Actually, there are very rarely tears, just a lump in the throat that one has grown skilled at getting rid of.

**05 Dec 66**   For some reason, the compound seems particularly restricting tonight. Without thinking, I find myself anticipating a walk (or a drive) and am brought back to reality by the realization that one is allowed to walk only within the compound or along the streets of Bien Hoa... Oh, yes, and of course, along the roads of other compounds, if there were those that we could visit. Glenn Yarborough on the tape… "sleep my love and dream as you do…"

I would so like to hop aboard one of the choppers. It would be some type of release, I suppose, just flying. Marlon Brando in the movie tonight. Mac suggested that we watch it. It's worth a try.

**20 Dec 66**   We did hop a chopper! Was it legal? Probably not, but I didn't dwell on the question. Timeline: Vung Tau on the coast, 2245. The room is cool. A light breeze from the window ensures this. The breeze also carries the strains of Venite Adoremus. The staff of the 36$^{th}$ Evac (here) is practicing Christmas carols. For the first time since arriving in Vietnam, I have experienced several hours of refreshingly cool air, a meal out, and a sufficient amount of sleep two nights in a row. Hardship tour? Only in the broadest sense of the word. We have one day off per week, and on work nights, I retire no earlier than on that one night, hence not enough sleep. The afternoon was spent on the beach; in a matter of two hours, enough sun was absorbed to yield a painful burn… all in all, these two days have been refreshing, not even the sound of artillery. The other night at Phu Loi, it'd like to shake one's teeth loose. This early a.m., someone slammed the door, and I started right out of sleep, believing it to be another explosion from the ammo dump.

One mishap today, a Vietnamese youngster came running up "mama-san, mama-san" with a variety of gestures and pointing to where Pat had left her uniform. Sure enough, the pockets had been picked of $50. Yes, it could've happened in New York or Chicago or anyplace else, but it happened here.

The kids otherwise play and smile and run like kids everywhere. Perhaps they don't realize their dilemma. One little fellow in particular, about 4 years old, with crude inadequate crutches and a spindle-like leg, which hangs motionless… and he smiles and looks up and asks, "Can you give me anything?" My mind reels… anything? Not my watch or some candy... like the others, but anything. We can give only things. Finally, I answer "NO" and turn away.

Evening now… peaceful to sit over coffee watching the deep rose sunset between the ships anchored in the harbor; this, the South China Sea. Sounds exotic. The Ninth Infantry Division arrived today, and their band is playing, of all things, Caissons… and Christmas carols. Peaceful, though slightly unnerving to walk along darkened streets; ironic to pass concertina wire and armed guards with the sound of Silent Night in the background.

"Hello, Yank." The soldiers pass. Somehow seeing troops from other countries (Australia) isn't inspiring. What price being a US ally, eh what? Even the carols do not move me. Perhaps my feelings have become saturated, and as I have learned not to succumb to tears or anger, I've sealed off feelings of tenderness as well. It's like being suspended in time here, no significance to a given day, just perpetual summer. The date becomes incidental, for it is as yet too soon to count how many days remain before leaving. Sometimes it seems that probably no one ever leaves.

**24 Dec 66 (1150)**   It's Christmas, even in the States. It's around noon there. The past few days have been busy with various activities finally catching up with me. The "collapse" occurred tonight about two hours ago. I can't remember ever being more tired. Armed Forces radio has erupted into pronounced sputterings and intermittent Christmas music. "This Christmas program is brought to you live from Camron Bay, Republic of Vietnam. We are waiting for Cardinal Spellman." The evening has been exceptionally quiet. Perhaps it's the result of the Christmas truce in effect since 0700 today.

Oddly, I will see Christmas day in alone. I was to attend church with Tam, Pat, Maggie and Mac. We are a closely-knit group of friends. Somehow, I fell asleep instead of getting organized and joining them. The radio continues with interviews of the troops, "Tell me SGT, what's it like in Michigan right now?" Michigan!… my home of record. I cried.

Christmas now! The last five evenings have been consumed visiting with Tony and caroling on the units tonight. I try not to resent the above loss of time. Tony is just in from the field and needs the company and the caroling, especially at the chopper pad. It was mutually beneficial. As a result, however, there's just too much left undone. I did get a few Christmas presents at the PX and have even been able to wrap them in time for our get-together later tonight.

I've been in Vietnam nearly 2 months now, and there has been more variety of experience in that time than perhaps in the past several years of my life. On occasion, the confinement within the immediate area has been frightening, though. One day I even started to walk across the road, past the ARVN (Army of the Republic of Vietnam) Unit and into a nearby field. It was foolish and dangerous and caused quite a stir. It's also difficult to sit by the chopper pad remembering my recent flight to Vung Tau and to experience again the odd exhilaration of scanning the countryside with an awareness of beauty and a vague uncertainty for the safety of the aircraft occupants. It has been difficult to hear a friend apologize for his dislike of "drawing fire" (Who wouldn't dislike that?) during dust-off missions. It is a lonely feeling to realize the total absence of one's loved ones.

But there have been remarkable examples of the human capacity to overcome, to extend compassion and share optimism. Such was our Christmas of 1966 and will remain so, inextricably bound to a TO&E (Table of Organization & Equipment) personified as the 93rd Evac.

The radio mass continues… "Lord God, Lamb of God, under God."

In August of 66, I joined the Army Nurse Corps. I was assigned to RVN (Republic of Vietnam), per request, in October of that year. It is now a new year.

A new year. As Capt. Monroe said yesterday, "…In the blessed year of DEROS." (Date of Estimated Return from Overseas). Sitting here luxuriating in the thought of sleeping in tomorrow. I've been feeling a little tired, what with the effects of the GIs (true to Lieut. Nolan's prediction) even a small sample of spoiled fish can have its devastating effects. I'm afraid she'll be disappointed in her prediction of mortality, however.

The fish was consumed as part of what had been intended as a New Year's Eve celebration. I got off work at 2315 and joined Mac for some music and popcorn. We had cokes too, (the first in a long time). Suddenly, we heard several sharp cracks. Soon the single shots gave way to increasing automatic fire, which seemed to be coming from all directions. We looked outside. Flares burned over the chopper pad, and we were not at all reassured by an unmistakable stream of incoming tracer rounds. "Oh Lord"—the hospital itself was under attack, and nearly everybody was at the club obtaining a liberal supply of liquor! I kept urging Mac to wear her helmet whilst we peeked from behind a makeshift barrier… "Soft tissue repairs itself," I cautioned; "the cranium not so much."

We were about to leave for our Units when Pat sauntered in. In the melee, we had overlooked what now seems obvious, it was 1215, and the taxpayers had just subsidized one hell of a New Year's celebration. It was 1 Jan 67.

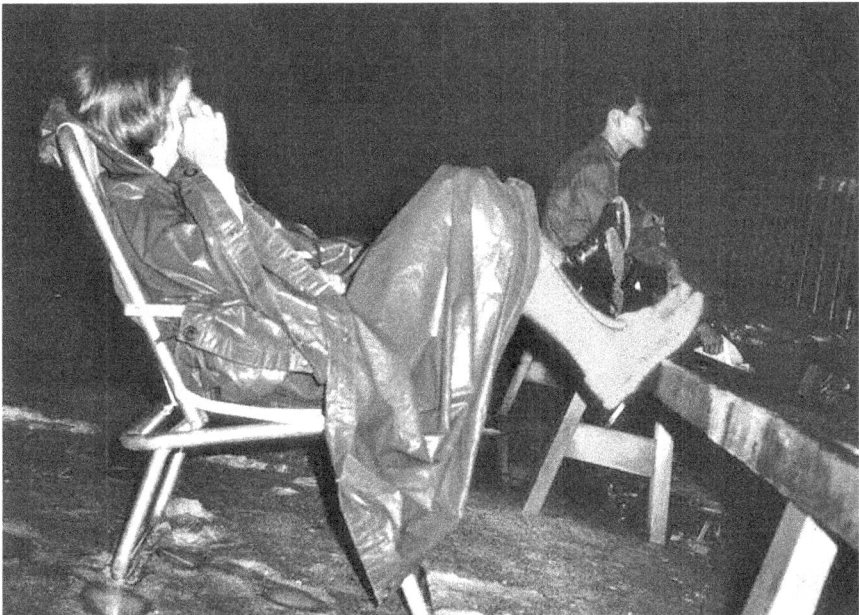

**The Nightly Movie**

Fay Ferington

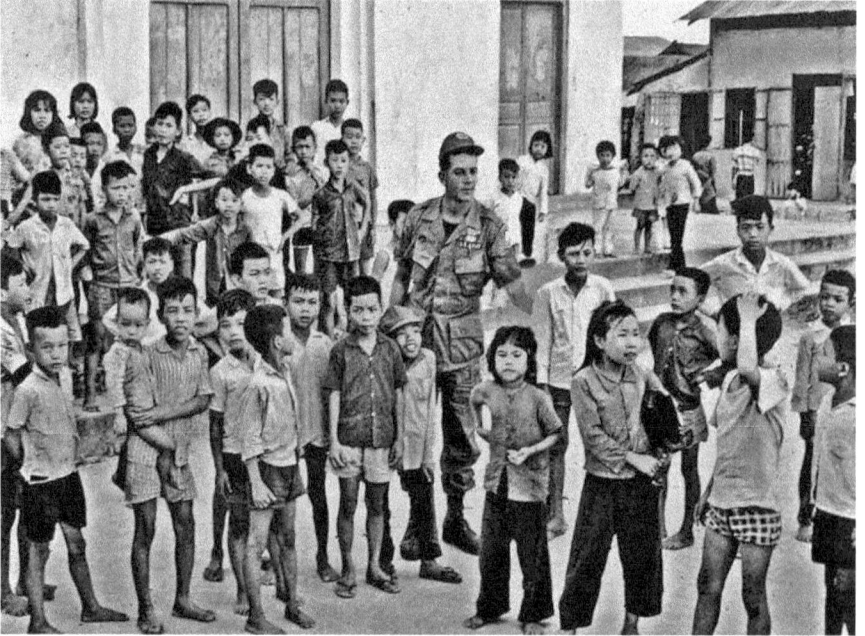

Medical Civic Action Program

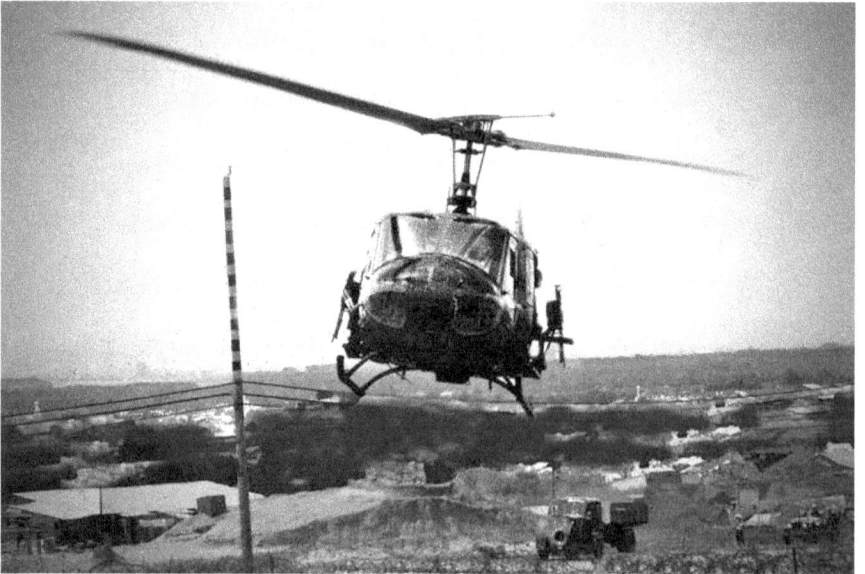

We Hopped a Chopper

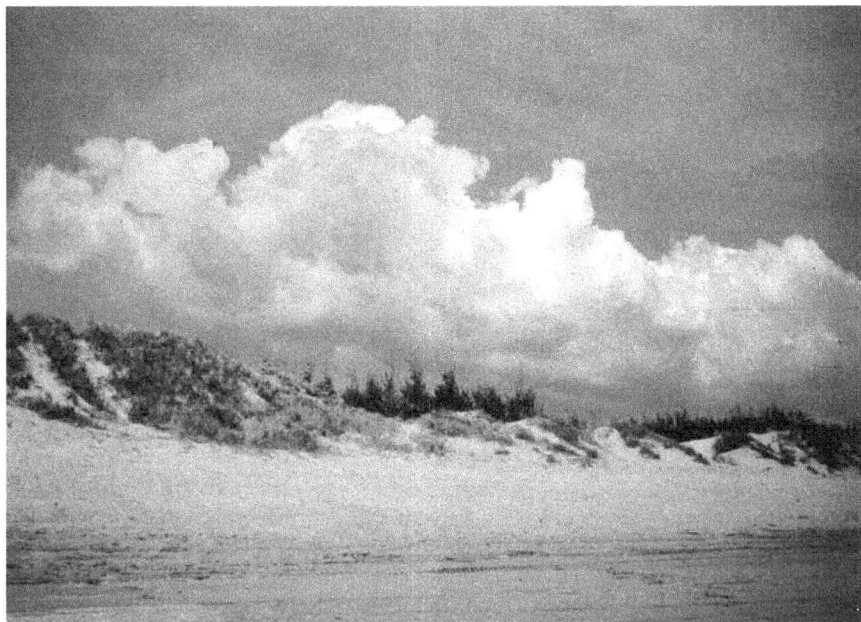

**Beach along the South China Sea**

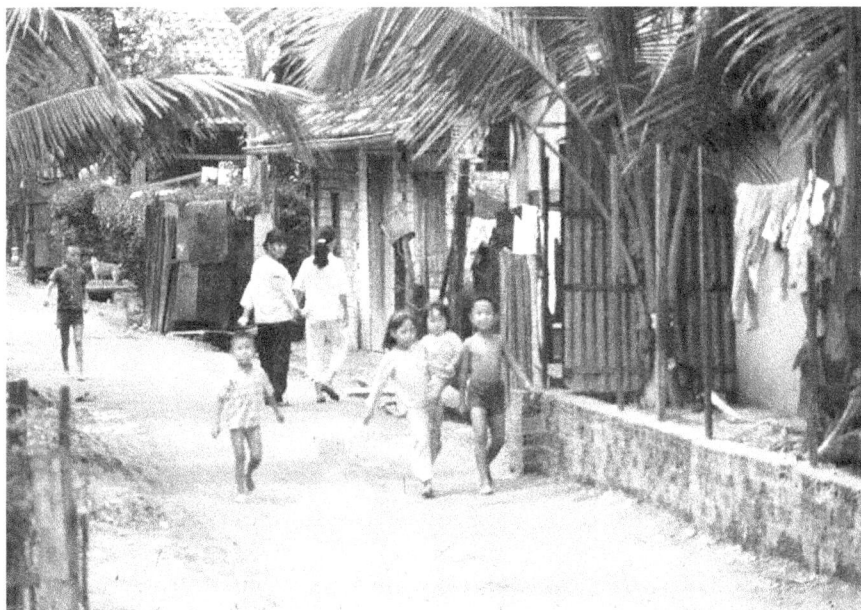

**Vung Tau Street Scene**

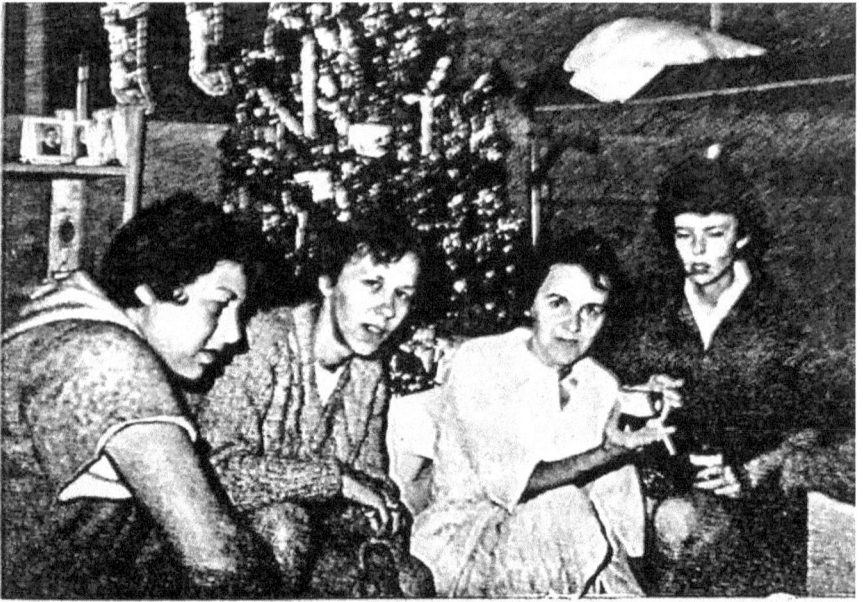

December 24, 1966    Republic of Vietnam

Pat, Fay, Tam, and Hawk (Mac took the photo)

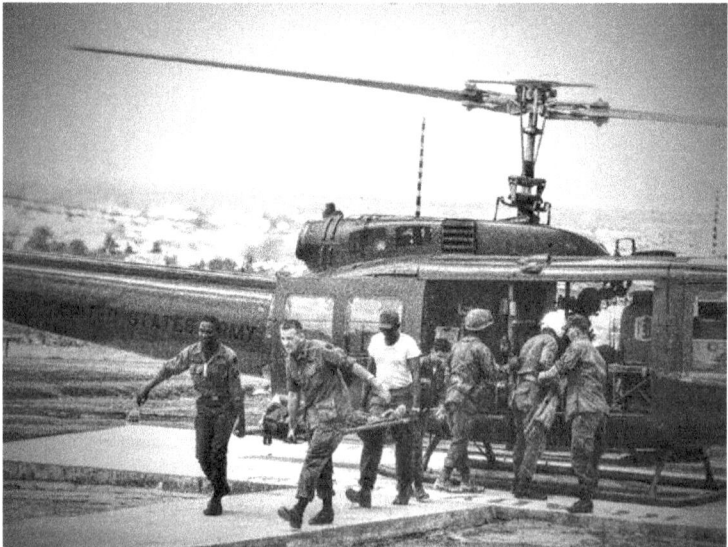

Evac Arrival

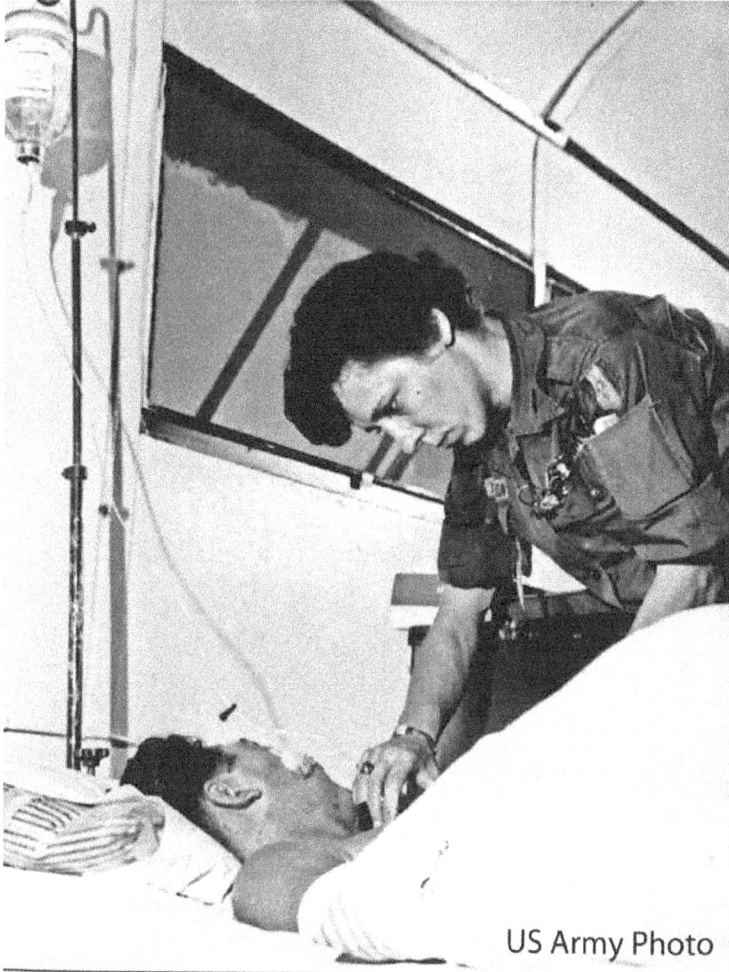

US Army photo

# Chapter 4: A New Year
# (03 Jan 67 – 30 Jan 67)

**03 Jan 67**   If we must have a war, how about having it right here? We sit high and dry, listening to stereo tapes, sleepy with the bulk of good food, with the effort to discover new variations of the day's luxury. We sit logy with the day's heat, only occasionally silent in recalling one man's pain. Hell, I'd rather be where the action is. Maybe there wouldn't be so much time to think.

**07 Jan 67**   On a lunch break. All AM, it's been a terrific rush, but mostly, I'm afraid, due to my own clumsiness. I took far too long to mix several IVs, to include adding Aqueous Pen and Terramycin to each. It's a good thing the noon meds were set up early. Sometimes I think the day will never come when I won't have to ask someone or check the PDR every time something is ordered, which I haven't done at least once since arriving in RVN. Over the hurtle today, though, and, in fact, it has been a rather appropriate challenge… the ward and back to med-surg, the Army and RVN all at once… WHEW!

**08 Jan 67**   We evac'ed 14 patients to the Vung Toa today, some weary of the intricacy of the Army medical service treatment network, some apparently delighted with the move. The afternoon was quiet, routine, and with a smile, Capt. W announced that we were to quote "empty" the ward. There was an operation, in fact, a big one, and we needed all beds available.

"Where was the operation? The Delta?"

"I don't know."

"How casually we seek classified information."

"The best way to stay out of trouble is not to know any."

Half hour later, 14 of our men left for A&D (Admissions & Dispositions), hopefully to board a CH 47 (chinook helicopter = chopper) to the 36th Evac (in Vung Tau). Fifteen minutes later, 14 men, the same, returned with word that A&D knew nothing of the evacuation.

Several phone calls later.

"Hang loose. If they don't go out tonight, they'll go out tomorrow."

Maybe they'll go out, and surely, they'll take their stories with them. That was yesterday. B with his memories of his wife and infant daughter.

W: "I don't want to go out there again. I've been here six months. That's enough. They should have a man rotate to a rear area after six months."

A: "I'd be scared to go out now; it doesn't bother you until you get hit; never bothered me before."

T: "Yeah, we're a few miles outside of Pleiku. You know we live in holes about that deep. The first day back there Charlie kept us in those holes all day." (And then he relates the fatal error of another unit and its subsequent casualties.)

W and A and T and even S with the smell of marijuana still on his clothing… men of average stature, with little relish for the experience of combat: "Hell, uh, heck, I'm U.S. (i.e., drafted) man!"

But they go, and they don't look back on the way out the door.

**11 Jan 67** Violence and more of the same. It's accepted rather casually. I suppose I better become more casual about it, also. Still only one admission from the Delta operation. It's been hectic, mood-wise, though. One of the psychiatry patients ran off the ward last night, was nearly shot by our own guards, made it through the gate only to get shot by the ARVN (Army of the Republic of Vietnam). He died today. A miserable epitaph.

**13 Jan 67** In rereading this log, I find moments when I felt pretty good, confident of my capacity to withstand the events of the next year. Probably because I've been able to control a tendency to daydream about those aspects of life which are more desirable. It seems possible to just "turn it off" in favor of supposedly trivial events each day—the use of a neighbor's hotplate, water for the evening shower, an orange for breakfast, a cold beer…

My shoulders ache. I really hated to start that blood this afternoon, the patient had been severely wounded, and now it's as if having become convinced that he was going to live, he has become fearful of the slightest discomfort. I certainly didn't want to stick him more than once. I adopted a most convincing bedside manner, and the needle went in.

BIG NEWS: We have been designated POW ward along with the two or three other types of services. There's Charlie, and in contrast to being big as life or fierce as the gaping wounds his weapons inflict, he's small and still. The tenacity with which he is rumored to cling to "the mission" would be called courage if he were other than VC (Viet Cong). I'm his nurse. I look into his eyes with conflict, and the ache across my shoulders grows.

**14 Jan 67** *After I had served as an army nurse for three months in Vietnam, I wrote the following questions. As I retyped these questions, nearly verbatim, fifty-plus years later, numerous responses occurred to me. These are provided at the end of each question.*

Upon departing CONUS (Continental United States) amid an array of farewell gatherings, a somewhat sagacious individual remarked, "Have a good war." Upon my return, a less wise person might ask, "How was it?" And I will say nothing of consequence but think, "you wouldn't ask if you could answer these questions." (Or… "If you could ever know.")

What is it like when you realize that… the environment you have chosen can be unpredictably deadly?

*("My God," the shrill sound of fragments passing near my shoulder might have ended everything?)*

What does one do when reporting for duty impressed with such knowledge?

*(…One heads toward the Unit rapidly and in a crouched position.)*

How much can one miss… his homeland?

*(…Her homeland.)*

Is it possible to long… for the sound of a horn or the opportunity to soak in a hot tub?

*(Or… for the chance to have any one less day in this country?)*

What does one do after discovering that an "enemy attack" … was a New Year's Eve celebration?

*(…Be glad that the tracer rounds were not aimed at you.)*

What… is the loudest sound you have ever heard?

*(…What does a pad of 10,000 artillery shells exploding several dozen times through the night sound like from a distance of 1/4 mile?)*

Do you or have you ever… lived in the vicinity of rats?

*(Or… checked your bed at night and tucked in the sheets to avoid a rat getting in with you?)*

How bright are surveillance flares... a mile away?

*(Or... 300 feet away, for that matter?)*

Can one mistake the slamming of a door for an explosion?

*(…In contrast, awakened by explosions one night, I went back to sleep thinking… it's only the war.")*

How does one converse over the sound of 105 mm howitzers?

*(...Especially when they're routinely fired over the building where you work?)*

How does the enemy behave while being cared for in confinement?

*(...Most are quiet and cooperative unless abused by the attitude or manner of a care provider.)*

Does every injury resulting from hostile action deserve a medal?

*(Or... Does any medal speak of an experience another can know, much less quantify?)*

What does one say to a man who, having lived in mud, with bugs and leeches and the hell of modern weaponry, asks why he must risk "going out" again?

*(...I only listened.)*

Should one not acknowledge (apologize) for the enjoyment of luxury?

*(...For the benefit of hot meals, a cot and sheets and a roof that only leaks a little bit, and only in a few places.)*

What does one do when casualty after casualty is being presented, and you can do so little?

*(...When for want of a critical assignment, you sit and <u>wait</u>, but in <u>immediate </u>awareness until you are needed... be it an hour, or a day, or as sometimes happens, not at all?)*

How does one best serve the needs of a friend, knowing that he may be injured or killed as a part of the routine course of events?

*(...Or one's self; I was at my next assignment, Texas, and ran into Herb one day. He had rotated a month or so after I did, and I ask, "How were Tom and the other guys when you left?" ...He said only, "Tom didn't make it.")*

**20 Jan 67**  We've been getting more seriously wounded patients lately (POWs). Sunday, one whole wing of the ward was set aside for post-op placement. We were not accustomed to the demands of so needy a population, and it took some real doing to shift gears. The wing is full now, as of yesterday. Several of the VCs (Viet Cong) are in hip spicas, one with an amputation in addition to the casts. Wednesday, we received two with fresh amputations. Their nutrition is generally very poor, as is their blood work. IV fluids and blood have been given liberally. Surprisingly, the majority eat our regular diets with no apparent problems. They warm up to being cared for with a readiness and are cooperative, except for one youngster who refuses to smile and is nonverbal. It's not possible to tell if this is due to hostility or depression.

One boy (he never grew a beard) sought reassurance several times that his leg would not be amputated. It is rumored that Vietnamese, as well as VC, amputate more often than not. I told him it would be saved. "GI medicine number 1." A foolish blunder on my part, for two days later, I sat with an arm around his shoulder while tears filled his eyes at the sight of his stump. His face was otherwise impassive. I gave him a cigarette and had one myself.

That same day, pictures were taken, which I assumed were for the purpose of propaganda. Maybe "that boy" is fortunate. He can neither be forced to rejoin his buddies nor can he volunteer for such. Later that afternoon, Ginny walked onto the ward. She was tired from the flight and taxed, I'm sure, by having driven through Bien Hoa to the 90th Replacement Center before arriving here, but she was the same warm, thoughtful person I remembered from basic.

**30 Jan 67**  The past few days have been busy and gratifying… a new nurse on the ward will lighten the workload considerably, and even orienting her has been a joy. She appears conscientious and has an apparent sense of humor and enthusiasm for life.

Had yesterday and today off! Sleeping in 2 mornings in a row is enough to inspire one. In addition, Herb and I spent Friday evening at

2nd Field Forces for the purpose of entertaining. We had hoped to have a type of hootenanny, but the men, though attentive, were apparently not in the mood to sing. At any rate, it went fairly well as we rendered several versions of "He's Got the Whole World In His Hands"… "You and me brother in his hands, the US Army in his hands… he's even got Charlie in his hands"… we continued.

Yesterday was a day to simply pamper oneself. I had a manicure, a shampoo and a haircut. The hairdresser fussed endlessly while he followed his assistant about my head. Lying outside later (120 degrees plus in the sun) and 84 interruptions...

"Are you keeping a diary?"

"No. A memoir."

"You want to remember this place?"

"No, I want to remember that I had a life before coming to Vietnam." (Loud laughter from the "audience.")

—No more interruptions.

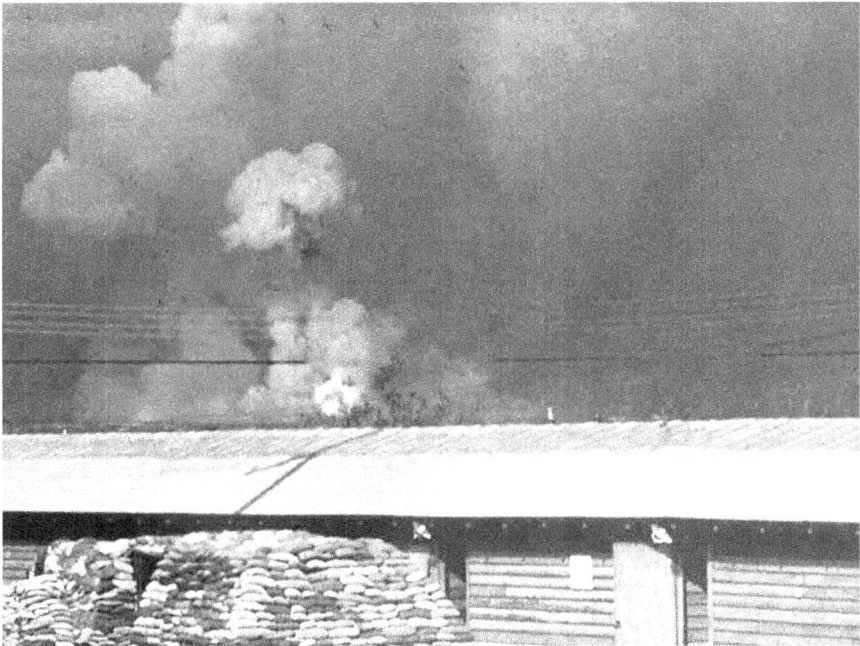

A Bombing?

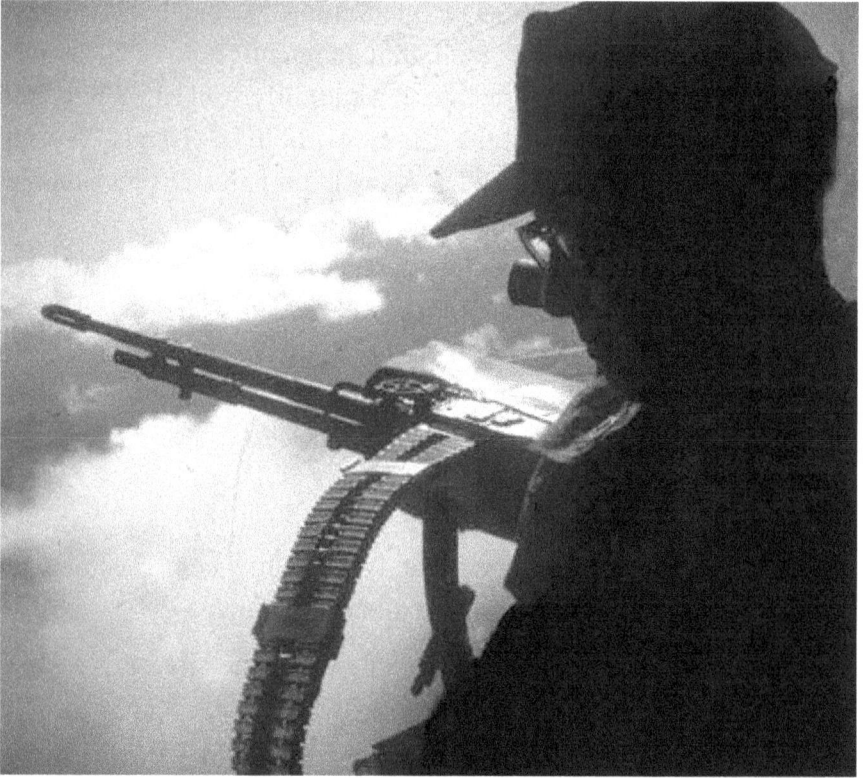

**The War Continues**

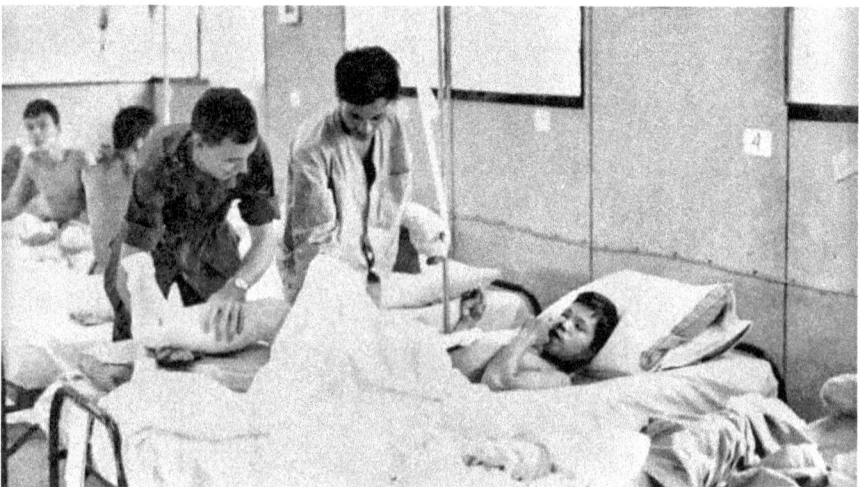

**Our medic Spec 4 C**

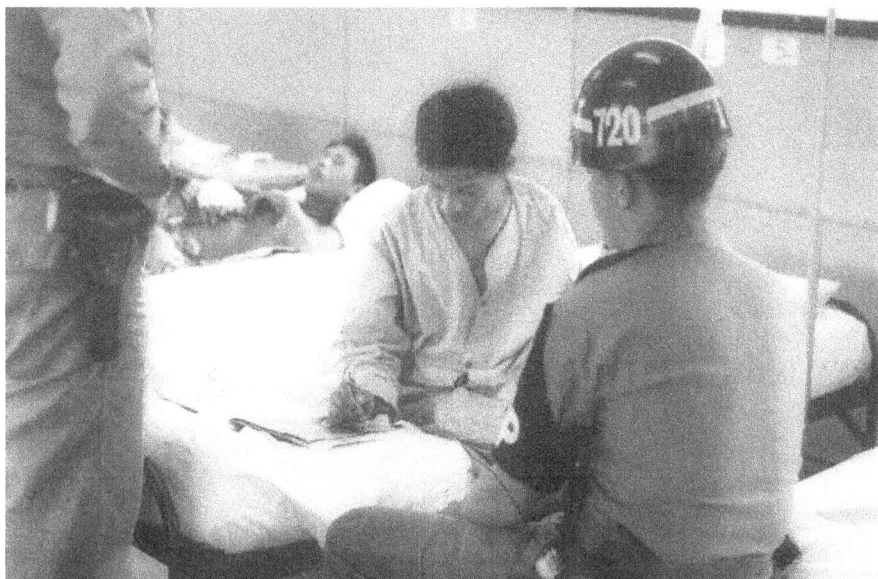

POW with MP

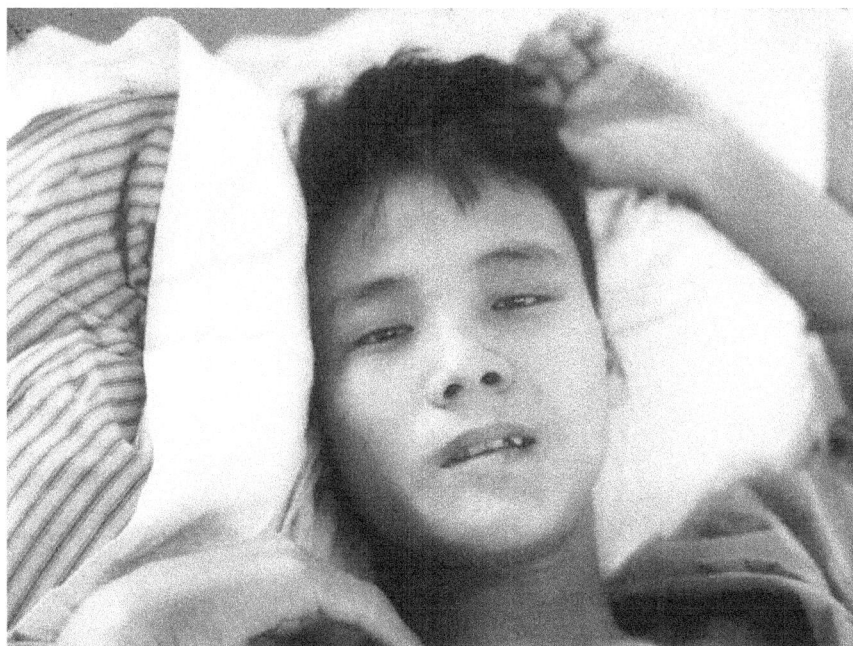

Phan Van Dia – a POW

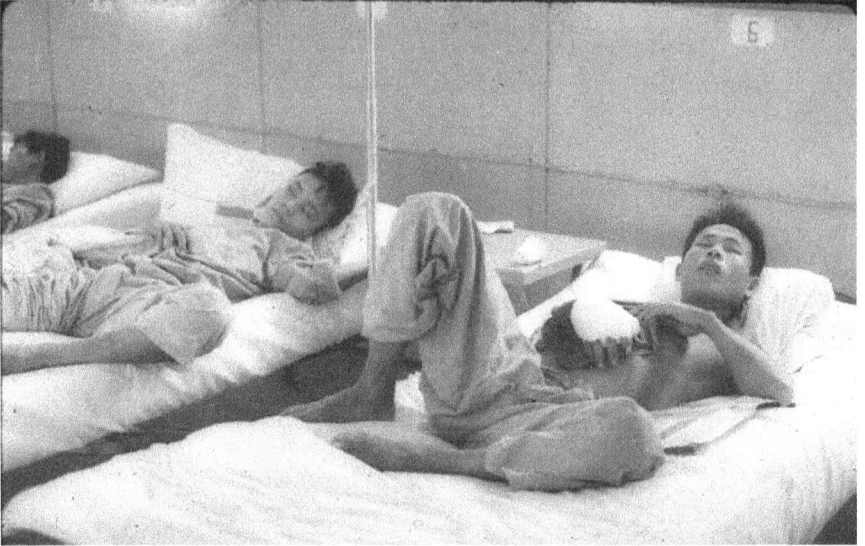

**Comfortable**

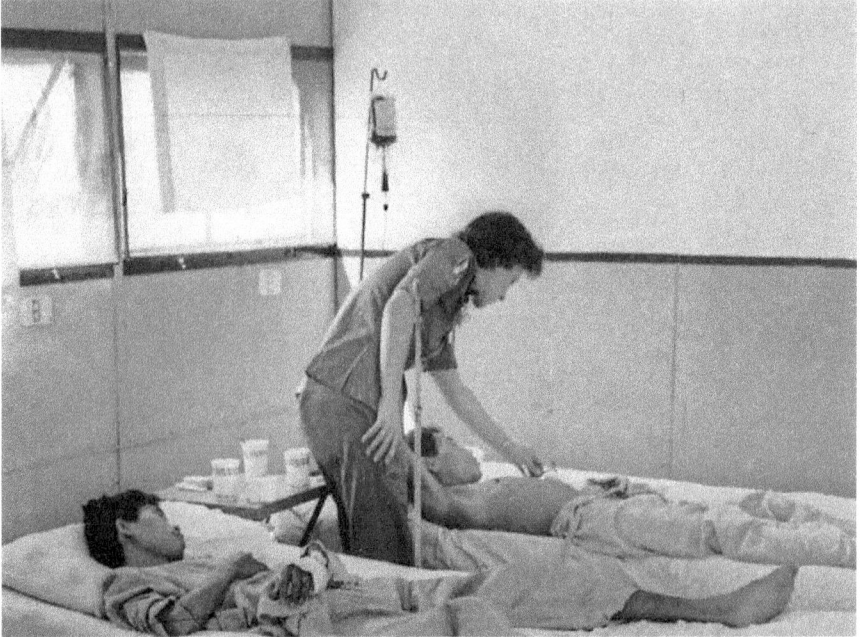

**Awaiting Surgery**

# Chapter 5: Close Calls
# (31 Jan 67 – 23 Mar 67)

**31 Jan 67** Midnight and one more time, I have completed a day and found myself seemingly without resources to arise in the morning… only, of course, I will. One more 5 minutes alone to reflect on the circumstances which would make one man want to scream (and indeed he did)… "I'm glad I got shot"… One more momentary awareness of the eternity we call a year. Awareness, followed by attention to trivia.

These are ludicrous circumstances… but, "I will live. I will live fully. I will not like all I see, but I will see it. Already I have seen a bomb explode against a tropic sky and gazed disinterestedly at the smoke beyond the palms"…

**04 Feb 67** Item #1 Time: 0245 …a very loud explosion, shaking the walls, awakened, I reach for my tape recorder to make sure that it rests secure on my bookcase… someone enters and leaves the quarters... It's quiet again. Sleep returns, and I dream of people at war with each other.

Item #2 Time: 0320 …a rapid and continuing succession of what in sleep first appeared to be small-arms fire. I awaken slowly this time and gradually realize that the sounds are exploding shells. I go outside to see what I can see and am greeted by a brilliant fire. The sky has become a great funnel-shaped cloud of smoke.

Item #3 Several others are up now, and bed lights are going on. A small group has gathered for the purpose of photographing the spectacle. Streaks of fire fly about. Large bursts punctuate the stream of smaller explosions. A few people wear their steel pots.

Item #4 Photographing the fire… another single resounding explosion sets off a new series of shells. I snap the shutter on an embroiled, rapidly ascending ball of fire, but at the nearby zing of what are apparently shell fragments, hasten to quarters and go to the bunker. The shells continue to go off, but after a while, it slackens to near silence.

Item #5 Time: 0500 I return to quarters. The fire is very localized now. It appears quite harmless. Then the bursts ignite pad after pad of ammunition, and the cycle is repeated.

Item #6 Time: 0600 A cup of coffee, a fresh uniform, it's almost time to go to work. I decide to tape some of the racket. It's surprising to play it back. It sounds more than anything like a drum-roll. The entire episode has become tiresome. Several people are angry. We estimate the cost to US taxpayers… a million dollars?… more? We really don't know. We go to work.

Item #7 Time: 0730 A phone call from HQ (Headquarters), "the next pad will produce a pronounced shockwave. We are expecting shrapnel." I speak with the patients. They are very calm. I've set up the next scheduled medications already; I turn out the lights and wait. At this time, a number of patients and staff sit on the floor between the beds. I wonder idly if the blast will scatter the meds. I wonder if there will be shrapnel. The chaplain sits there with us and remarks, "I've never been calmer."

Shortly the XO (executive officer) enters. He's agitated and urges us to be ready to evacuate the patients. Shortly, he says why. There is danger of exploding chlorine gas. Evacuate them where? Masks have been issued to a wing of the ward occupied by a signal corps outfit. It would be nice if there were some for us.

After about 45 minutes sitting there, the all-clear call comes through. We joke as the routine of the day is resumed. I found that bit about shrapnel hard to believe anyway. The Drs and I make rounds, but the explosions preclude any discussion, even though we're standing next to each other. We inspect various wounds anyway.

Item #8 Time: 1000 It's very quiet now, except for a few red and green flares going off. Actually, were not such violence implied, it would be quite lovely. At last, I leave the ward to go to the latrine, get as far as the rear door of quarters and am blown back several feet. Something sharp hits my face; sand, I assume later. One hears glass breaking, notes the shaking of the building and the dust. Someone calls out loudly, "Get to the bunker!" I reply reflexively, "I'm on duty, ma'am!" and leave for the Unit.

By 1130 the secondary explosions have nearly died out. I take a long lunch hour. In quarters those sleeping are still in their fatigues. Several are sleeping under their beds.

Item # 9 Time: 1400 A young Vietnamese girl enters the ward. She holds out her hand to reveal the name "Tony" written there. We have no one by that name. I apologize. She smiles and leaves. I think about "Tony" and the explosions. I wonder if he wrote his name on her palm... while the day resumes without further incident.

**08 Feb 67**    Time: 0430 Working nights and have just hit the 0400 slump. It's good that we resume a little activity shortly, or I'd probably just fall out of the chair.

Yesterday, the 1,600th patient was admitted to the 93rd since its arrival in RVN in the fall of '65. I notice some of the patients' numbers tonight were already up to the 60's past that mark. Tomorrow we will gain a few beds by evac'ing a half dozen people. Right now, the Unit census is 62. (Boy, what I'd give for a bed!)

**12 Feb 67**    This is a night, feelings about which I will not be proud. Man courts death and is fearful of his success. I feel like screaming out the insanity of our existence. The overt serenity around here is unnatural. I slept three hours after coming off duty early, attended a hail and farewell for our COs (commanding officers) and already feel so extraordinarily tired.

Earlier, I was awakened by a number of magnificent bursts. It develops that a minefield has been found, just inside the gate, just to the right of the main walkway. "Our team" was detonating such in accordance with progress. A tank was called in. It had a big blade on the front of it, and it was driven around the area until all was safe. I counted 13 explosions. They were antipersonnel mines. Doesn't anybody realize that we could have crossed that same place at any time but, at the same time, we are refused opportunities to leave the Long Binh area because of surrounding "hostile" activity? To quote a friend who isn't allowed to join her fiancé nearby, "I'd rather be dead than lonely."

**19 Feb 67** A most peaceful day today... two patients to surgery, discharged five, leaving the lowest census we've had, ever.

In anticipation: R&R coming up the first week in April. It should be spring in Japan. How lovely it will be to see grass, newly opened leaves, flowers and people involved in the everyday activities of living. I really don't expect to feel part of it all though. Perhaps inadvertently, this little war (if there is such a thing) has become the central point of our existence.

**23 Feb 67** Tomorrow is the tenth day at work, and by taking Saturday off this week and Sunday off the next, one gains 2 days in which to sleep in. Saturday will be a late breakfast consisting of 1) juice, 2) hotcakes and 3) coffee, all gloriously homemade on Shirley's hotplate; then it will be possible to hit the Air Force PX. Maybe they'll have Winstons!

Sunday afternoon, I'll try MedCap again. Dr. Marron says he's starting at an orphanage near Saigon. As opposed to previous endeavors, we shouldn't have to worry about the VC getting the medications, about civilians exchanging pills because they prefer a different color or about the difficulty of providing treatment in the absence of any records. For myself, it won't be necessary to play Dr. I'll concentrate on the children. It almost sounds optimistic. Monday, we'll go to Saigon to set up a clinic.

It's getting very warm these days. Ninety-six in quarters in the evening. Currently, though, down to 84 and quite comfortable. Tonight, we scrounged up some hot chocolate by means of a packet of such from "Maggie's Storehouse" and combined it with a can of whatever kind of milk they sell in the PX. I even found some Lorna Doones in the wall locker, though purchased in November, they were not unreasonably stale, and being in the locker, the mice and rats had not had access to them. (They've been in everything else, including some graham crackers and an apple I had put up on the bookcase.)

The monotony of having few patients to care for might well end shortly. Of course, that's unfortunate for others. The 11th Cav and the 173rd Airborne moved out last week (or was it a few days ago?). At any rate, they're catching hell up near the border... maybe dishing out a little too. Read in 10 Feb *Washington Post* of the expanding riots in Peking. It sounds very bad. I find it impossible to imagine one's homeland in such havoc. Thank God for the USA.

**25 Feb 67**   It is 0445. I have made general rounds two times tonight. All is exceptionally quiet in the house. I am tired. The first night is always more difficult. I have written 2 letters and am afraid that they will reflect a certain indifference.

Last night the artillery was slightly louder. A fervent wish to express my revulsion at the monotony and heat and confinement achieved some vicarious satisfaction with each explosion. "Give 'em hell" and the pre-fab walls shudder but not nearly enough to dislodge the two bugs crawling toward my bed.

Tam says I expect too much of people; says it's unfair to expect them to attain my level of performance. Could she ever understand how inadequate I feel that level to be? Probably not, and I shall not tell her. Far safer to withdraw ever so slightly... but without the old remorse and self-recrimination. Remember Mac's words, "You're too concerned with what others think of you."

Out of the contradictions, I seek consistencies to be bound together, yielding clues for appropriate response. One is a contradiction as one is uncertain. Who are you? What are you? I am random fibers seeking one another only tell me where my other colors lie.

Another page or two in the log. Another day or two in my life, recorded at first self-consciously, then with self-indulgence… a year of impressions and a record to insure insight into the effect of the environment upon this organism. How narrow a view of a circumstance the proportion of this, when young people are dying, when minds are stretched beyond their point of elasticity. What a predicament we are all in and what an anesthetic.

**28 Feb 67**   Mag is married! She took R&R in Hawaii and met Jerry (a Dr. formally assigned here), and they were married last Tuesday.

Jim is back from the field. Did the 173rd pull back? Not likely. I'll get some info on that soon enough.

We're losing two people from the ward. Rose is going to pre-op (where the expression "war is hell" loses its amusement value) and Matthews (clinical technician) is being pulled for 90 days TDY (temporary duty) someplace. "I guess we can't argue with the Department of Army." No, but I'd be willing to try. Sure hate to lose two such fine individuals.

**04 Mar 67**   On Taking a Lambretta Ride

This morning we went for a Lambretta ride (a 3-wheeled motorcycle conveyance). It cost 20 pi (piasters). We went from the hospital to the 90th Replacement Center, and the driver tried to argue with us about his fee. I told him to "take it and like it," all in a jovial tone, assuming that not knowing English, he could take no offense at the comment. I, in turn, gained some fiendish pleasure from guiltlessly so addressing another human. Of course, the price had been agreed upon before the journey had commenced. This agreement is SOP, for rates vary in direct proportion to the naiveté of the passenger.

The above procedure can be maddening, but in fact, should not be. In its most elementary form, it is a game and no more or less absurd than the multitude of games played in western cultures. The Lambretta driver plays at being offended that his fee is only that which one gives him. Presumably, the passenger should play at astonishment at the fee. The fact that both parties have previously agreed to that amount is an irrelevant observation. One might correctly haggle and hassle and resolve the matter with slightly additional compensation, having considered that additional compensation when estimating the fee in the initial exchange. Apparently, games are an integral part of one's culture. To be unfamiliar with the culture is to be uncertain of the rules of the game. Unfortunately, such frustration is most likely to yield anger, particularly toward that individual who forces your participation…

**05 Mar 67** They come to this room. They come for identification and for the purpose of being pronounced dead. They come to be cared for as well... to be healed, this room with its concrete floor and harsh fluorescent light... they come here, and it is cool and dry and welcoming.

The room is nearly empty now. It is 0100. A steel pot (helmet) lies discarded in one corner, a bottle of insect repellant tucked securely in the headband. An M-16 rests against a chair. The weapon has been cleared. On the floor is a small olive-drab bag with a piece of paper pinned to it… James, Pfc.

Outside here are boots. They are muddy and smeared with blood. There are no pairs. Seven who came here tonight are described simply as "KIA" (Killed In Action). Their recent presence duly noted in the evening report. It is quiet. One can hear the clacking of typewriters in A&D (Admissions and Dispositions) and the sound of the hospital's generators. On the pad, a helicopter is warming up. The room has been cleaned and restocked. It waits to be of service again, as it most assuredly will be. It waits, for that is all it can do.

**14 Mar 67**   My God… we have spent Thy Grace…

**15 Mar 67**   Already halfway through the month. Why was it February dragged so? Ten days since 5 Mar 67.

**20 Mar 67**   Five months ago today, we left Travis Air Force Base. Twenty-eight days from today, we (Mac, Mag, Tam, Pat and I) will report to Camp Alpha in preparation for 7 days in Japan.

Last Friday, we moved into new quarters, an H-shaped building, tropical, 15 living areas per wing, 8 by 12 each with a 30-inch-wide screen at the top and bottom, the length of each… communion with the great outdoors!

There are a multitude of luxuries here. There is running water, there are sinks and private partitions between living areas. There is a lounge that is air-conditioned. The first night after packing and unpacking for several hours, we were a pretty grimy crew, and it was almost strange to just walk a few feet down the hall to clean up. Eventually, the water will be potable and hot. That should do something for our complexions. We flushed a toilet Friday also!

The dust of late is nearly beyond description. The first 2-inches of ground is a fine white powder shifted by such profound forces as the pressure of a footfall. The guys are filthy when they come in from the field, and we aren't much cleaner. This remarkable dirt blows liberally through the screened areas that make up the walls of the quarters. One should clean the area daily, but that would preclude the completion of other essentials.

Tonight has turned into a most pleasant experience. Pat is reading (on her bed); Mac is sitting against the bed listening to "Funny Girl" on the earphones and I'm writing this leaning against the wall locker. The paper said as of March 4th, we passed a week of the highest casualty count thus far. Apparently, the number of medical facilities in the area engenders an obverse impression. We have not been busy lately. Ran into Jonny yesterday. He's left the 1st Division and is a pilot with some helicopter assault unit. He spoke depressingly of several deaths, of problems with ship maintenance, but still of his desire to "extend" (add 6 months to his tour). He has no wife or family. Perhaps that's why he thinks this way—he has a couple purple hearts already.

**23 Mar 67** To paraphrase: "Dust, dust everywhere;" in one's nose and throat, streaking one's saliva. It covers the sheen of one's hair and clogs one's pores while sleeping. It blows like snow; it is white and without texture. Ah, for the mud of the rainy season. Twenty-four more days until R&R.

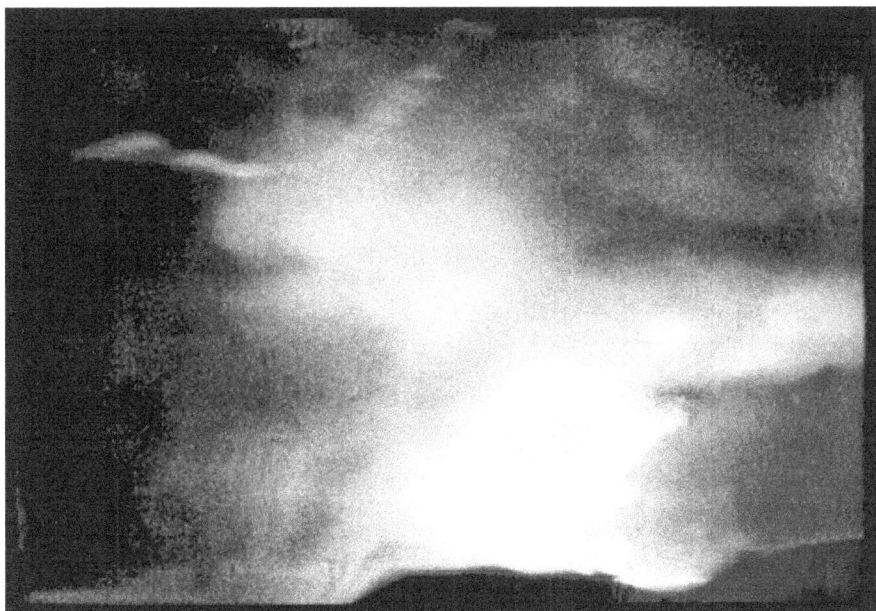

**Height of Attack**

Fay Ferington

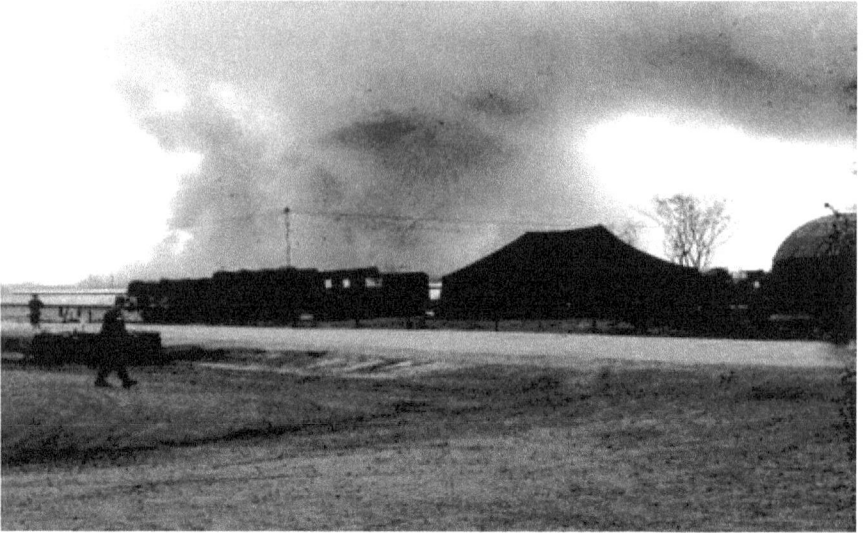

Morning -- finally!

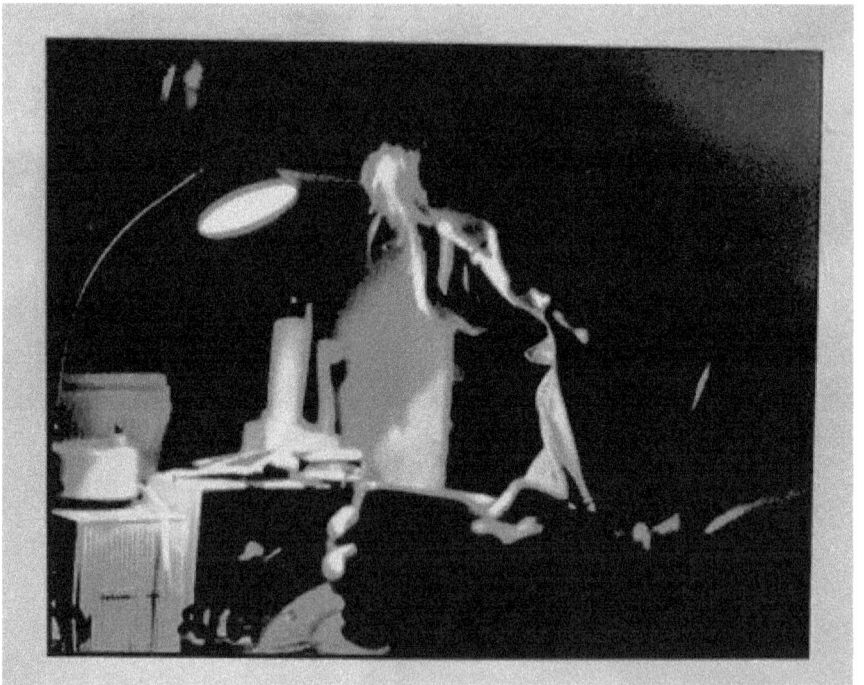

Mac Has Coffee Before Work

62

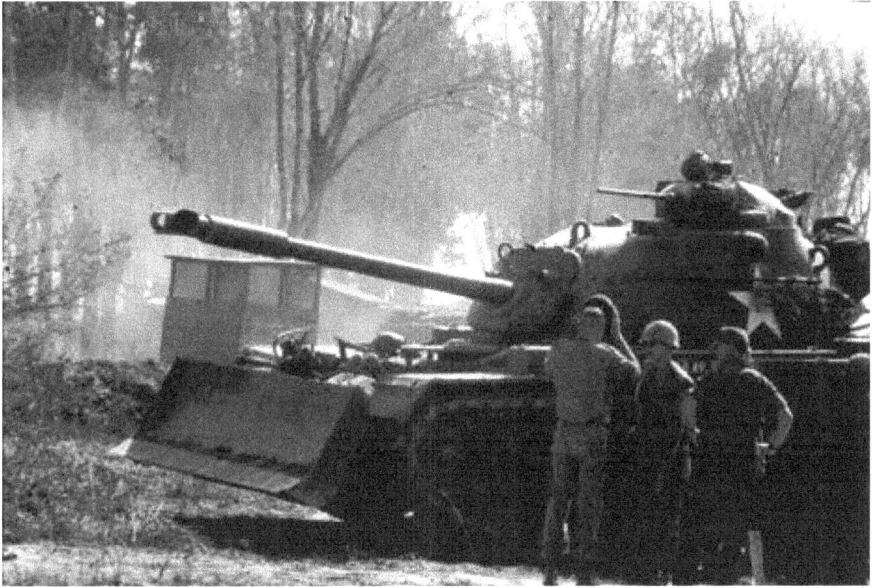

Clearing Anti-personnel Mines

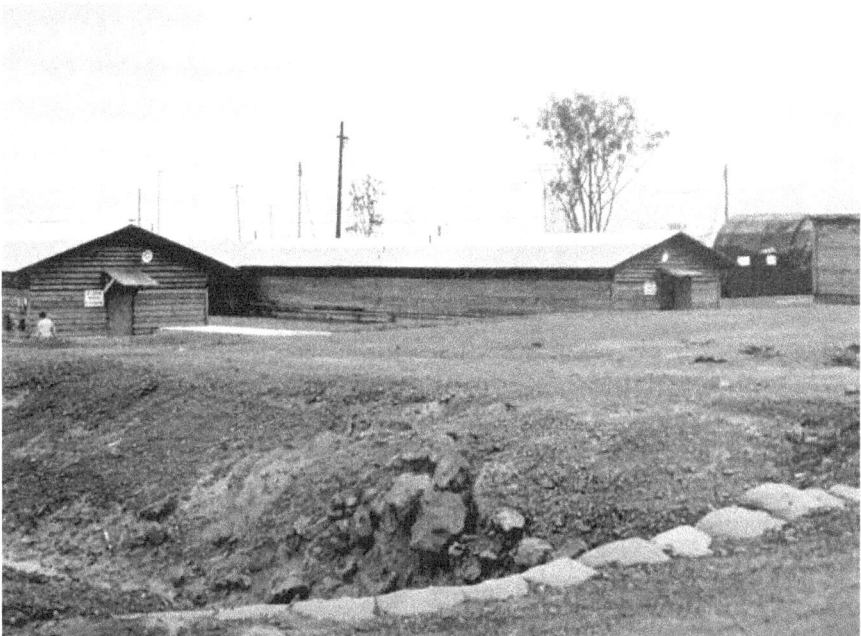

Our New BOQ

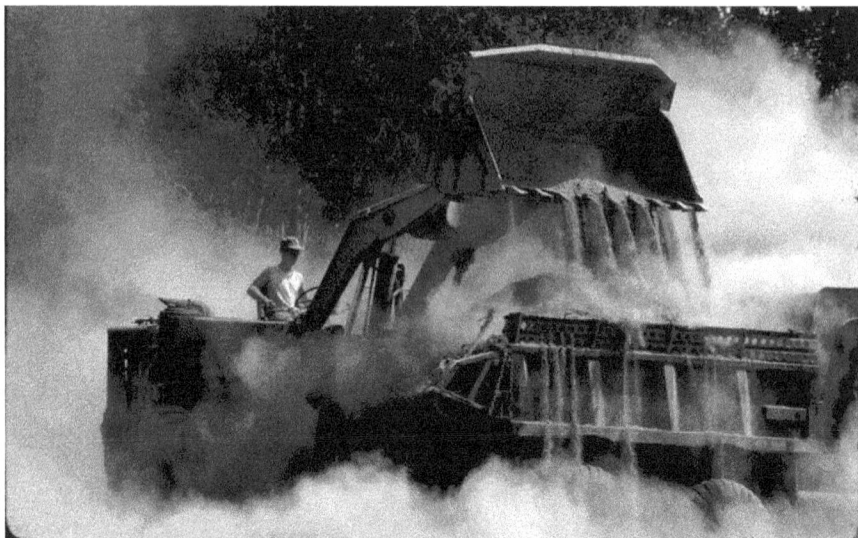

**The Dry Season**

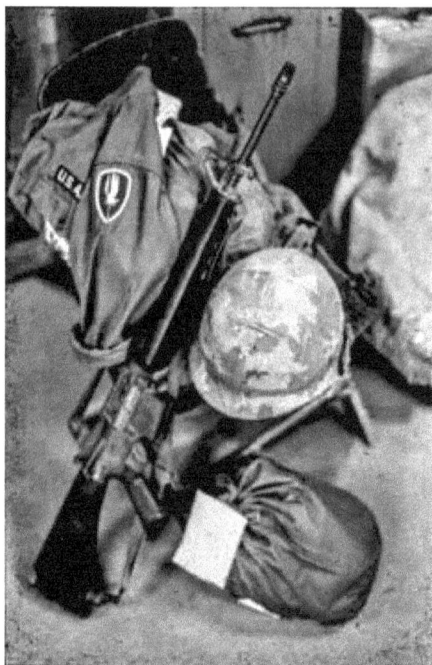

**Some Belongings**

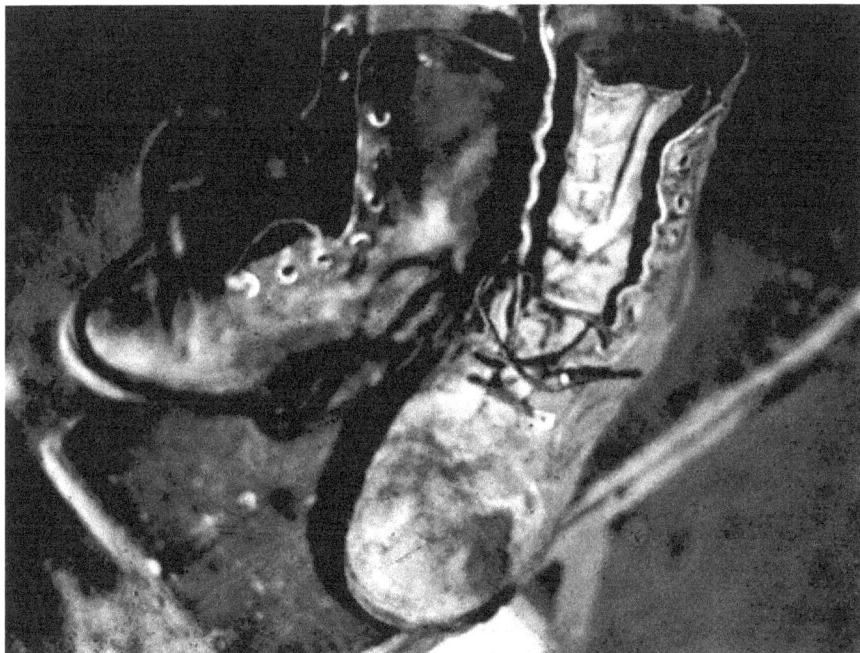

One Man's Boots

# Chapter 6: A Change of Pace
# (28 Mar 67 – 26 Apr 67)

**28 Mar 67** Had a small panic attack this morning after walking on the ward to discover the 1st premature infant I've seen in 9 years. She must be tough as leather to have lived to the ripe old age of about a month. Dr. Hill found her at the orphanage at Bien Hoa. She weighs 2.5 pounds. We padded a cardboard box, warmed it with a light bulb, and ran in oxygen using a rolled-up paper cup to direct the flow. She is gavaged every 3 hours, suctioned with a #8 catheter, using 10cc syringe. She is medicated per tube q6h, turned q2h and diapered with a cotton ball. One slaps her feet to obtain lung-expanding exercises, commonly referred to as crying. A rash on what will become her "bottom" is clearing nicely, but she has some degree of atelectasis in her left lung.

Perhaps as heartwarming as the pink in her nailbeds is the sight of one brawny paratrooper hovering on the periphery, occasionally murmuring to no one in particular—fascinating… just fascinating.

**04 Apr 67** The baby died today at 1645. She went into heart failure. I should have anticipated it but hadn't really.

**07 Apr 67** It has been a busy week. Last Friday and Saturday, Drs. W and T did 43 cases between them. Our census jumped to 67 Sunday morning. We evacuated 25 to 3rd Field the same day, though. Casualties, about 25, came in yesterday, and the surgery beds are filling up again.

We received another child from the orphanage today. They say that he's a little over 4 years of age, is 29 inches long and weighs 15 pounds. He has a mild pneumonia, a marked strabismus and a maculopapular rash over his entire body. He's mute. He doesn't walk or indeed move much at all. He doesn't feed himself. He's supposedly toilet trained. His name is Taum.

**13 Apr 67**   How tragic that all life is to be, more often becomes what might have been. Often, it is that which is left unsaid which is most meaningful.

However, a progress note on Tommy:

1.   …eating a regular diet, gaining no weight

2.   …last Tuesday began making assorted sounds… among others "Da-da," a cry that sounds rather like a growl.

3.   Monday or Tuesday, he laughed, and Wednesday, after a couple of days, extended his arms to be held and later grasped a bedrail and pulled himself to his feet. When being held, he now snuggles up and drops his head against the other person.

4.   The skin lesions have nearly disappeared. Initial doses of piperazine resulted in his passing huge quantities of roundworms (approximately 12 ounces thereof, some up to 18 inches long). It wore him out. He slept most of today.

5.   …blood morphology …assorted sizes of hypochromic RBCs, and Dr. S. feels he's no doubt in need of vitamin B. His diet will be supplemented accordingly. His stool reveals some occult bleeding.

6.   He has an IVP tomorrow.

All in all, he's making rapid progress.

We were to go on leave this past Saturday. There are no R&R flights with vacancies until Tuesday. I'll believe it when we're in the air headed in a northeasterly direction. It rained briefly three times last week, and people were rooting for more. It has been 5 months since it last rained.

Heaven knows what the temperature has been lately, hotter than ever. Previously, one was not troubled until around 1100. By 0830 this past week, one could sit quietly and still ooze perspiration on one's face and neck. Artillery just started (2330). It's been quite close and frequent again this past week.

**16 Apr 67** Twenty-seven casualties (4 KIA, 23 WIA) when the 11th Cav Convoy stopped overnight at a PX at 11FF (2nd Field Forces). That's about a mile down the road… a secure area.

**17 Apr 67**   Tomorrow in Japan…

**26 Apr 67**   Japan was so good. How it points up what little things make one's life pleasant. We left the 93rd about 1100 on the 18th. A little way down the road, we saw large areas of smoke and flares. Closer to Saigon, heavy artillery exploded several times to the left of the highway. It made me anticipate leaving even more. Perhaps it should have given pause, but getting away from the continual air of violence seemed of primary importance. Tonight, I feel nostalgic. I wanted to resume work but can't say I was eager to return to the irritations and isolation here.

In Japan, there were pine trees and clean water flowing briskly over rocks. There were pink flowers and grass of so pure a green. There was snow on mountaintops and, one day, a brief episode of flurries. The air was cool. It felt so fine to breathe it deeply… it smelled fresh.

We saw thousands of cars and the large busy harbor of Yokohama. We saw taxicab drivers in white shirts and ties. We saw a real tulip on the dinner table. There was hot water. We visited a Japanese home with an exquisite garden. There were people who hadn't seen war in over twenty years.

The rains are trying to get started. It was raining when we landed yesterday morning. The baggage room at Tan Son Nhut was unchanged.

The rubble of Saigon was the same, and at 0800, the heavy, humid air was the same. This must be one of the most miserable countries in the world.

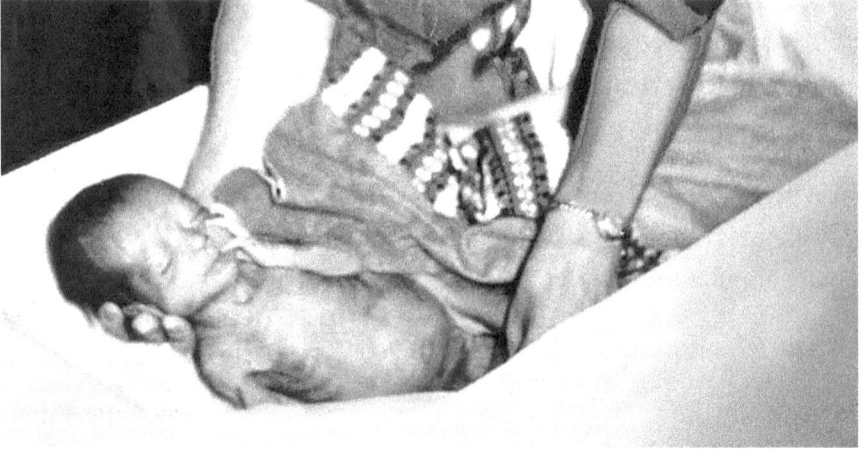

**Preemie**

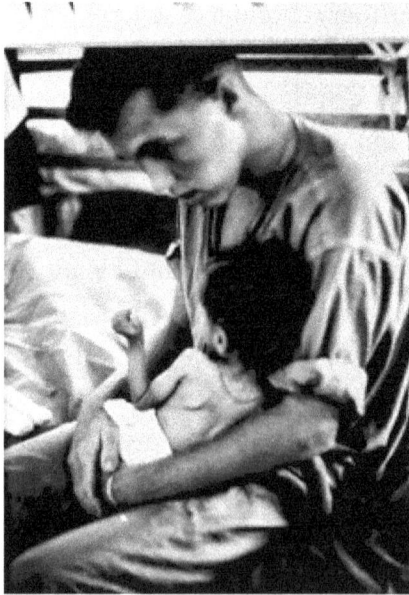

**Taum on Admission**

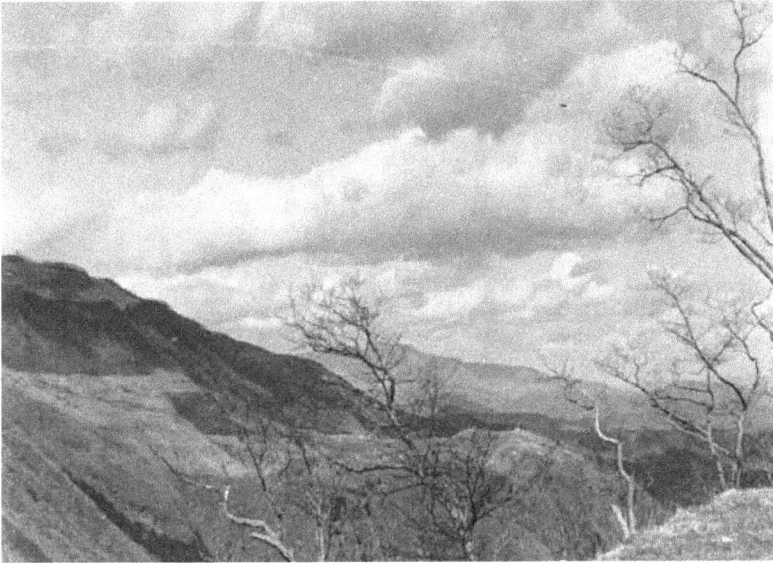

Japan 1

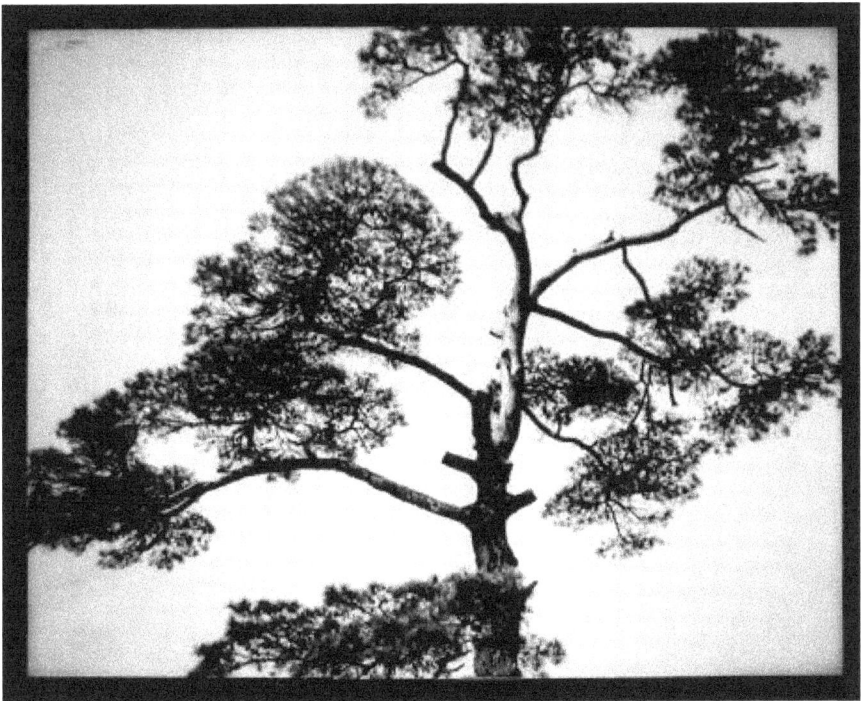

Japan 2

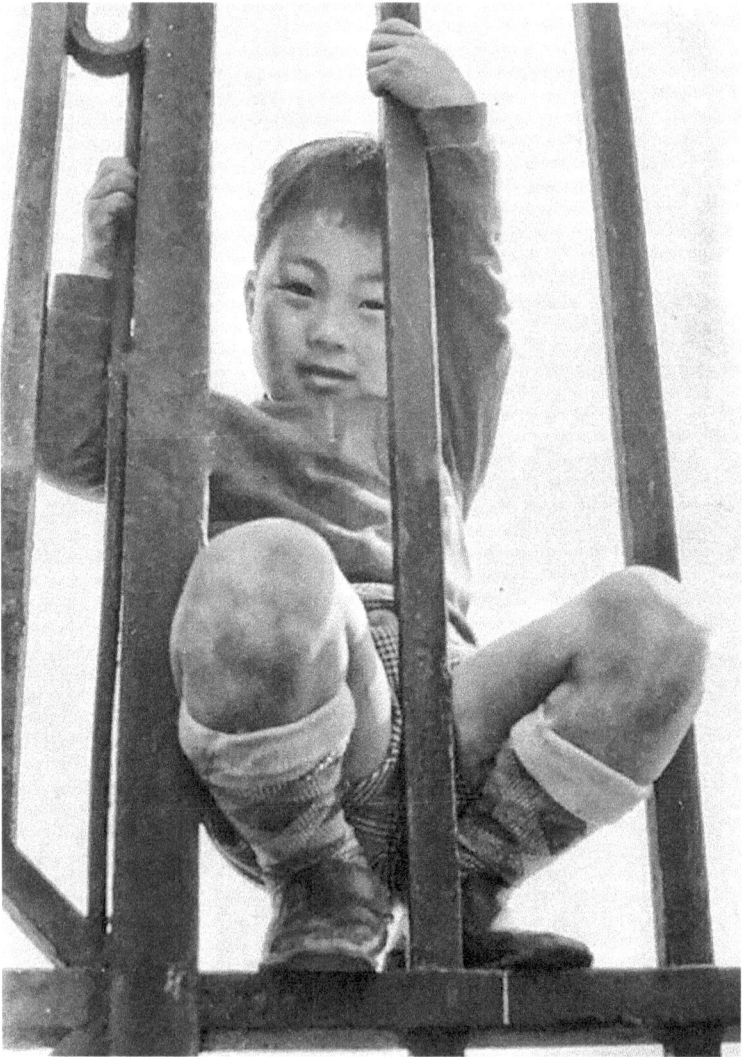

Japan 3

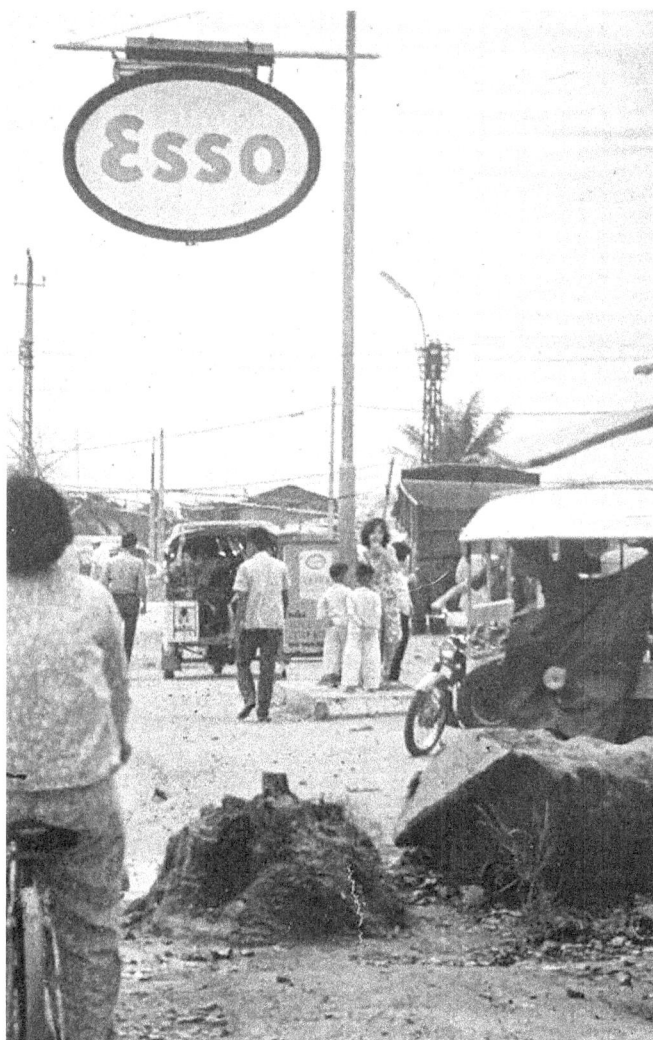

**Back in Saigon**

# Chapter 7: Questions
# (02 May 67 – 30 May 67)

**02 May 67**  I've scattered cups about the room to collect the rain coming in through our "new" roof… and it is raining! It's as though nature is compensating for the past months of dryness in one grand effort. Last Saturday, having obtained a paint brush from unit supply, I set about changing brown wallboard walls into three white and one "charcoal." The charcoal, incidentally, is that color referred to in military parlance as "battleship grey." It will be enhanced via an order placed with Sears Roebuck and Company: a gold spread, assorted colors of scatter pillows and a red wicker wastebasket. (The cup on the nearby bedside stand was placed incorrectly, and I now have an ashtray full of rainwater.)

Yesterday, Phyllis and I dissembled the bookcase and created a new look: a Danish entertainment center. This with the aid of a portable power saw from the orderly room, a T-square from some concerned male observers (who asked if we minded that they were watching us) and a bit of perspiration. Tonight, it was time to get rid of the VN dresser (a holdover from the old quarters). Pat was to lend a hand in disposing of it, but the rain precluded same, and there it sits in the corner. Ah well...

Progress Note on Tommy: He now weighs 18 and 1/4 pounds. His skin is completely cleared, he does knee bends ad lib, feeds himself, uses the "potty," makes "sounds" according to his wants, scoots alongside beds by holding on to the sheets, and laughs delightedly when tossed into the air. It is no longer possible to complete paperwork while he sits on one's lap. He grabs the papers, the pencil, your hand. Dr. McClure is so impressed with his progress that he feels he might soon be able to tolerate an anesthesia in order to do corrective surgery on his eyes. Currently, his right eye is patched in an effort to evaluate his vision in the other eye.

(If it rains like this all night, it will be interesting in the morning. Fortunately, everything is either covered with plastic or hidden away in the wall locker.)

Bedtime Ritual (2200): Shower again. While just sitting, writing, perspiration oozes from the backs of one's hands. It creates an unnatural sticky warmth. Turn back the poncho liner (bed cover) and sheet and place the fan so it blows across the opened area, eliminating the dampness. Prepare a uniform for tomorrow (ID, bandage scissors and hemostat in the shirt pocket; comb and cigarettes in various other pockets, blousing garters and socks in the boots... hang up the whole works... spray the room with insecticide to discourage the bugs that get in. They're not nearly as bad as they were last fall when they were so thick that one continually slapped at them in vain.

Into bed: Tuck in the edges of the sheet in case the rat that was on Mag's bed the other night pays a visit here... sink back. The mattress is soft. What the guys in the field would give for sheets and a bed like this... and a shower. (The rain is still pelting fiercely on our steel roof and dripping in in several different places. Too soon to tire of it, though. It cools things off, as long as it lasts anyway... no more dust (or rather sand)... sleep.

A loud, repetitive rumble; someone calls out, "Was that outgoing?"
"Yep."
"That's thunder. No, really, it was thunder."
I hope the lights don't go out tonight. Ever since that guy hid in the chief nurse's area and attacked her... I fall back to sleep.

Awake again. It's not thunder this time. Resounding whacks. Outgoing? Who cares? I went to bed to get some extra sleep. It's almost 0200. It's very quiet. No sound from the generator; the lights are out. Some flashlights bounce around down the hall. The rain is still "rattling the rafters" and still dripping in… damn.

<u>0600</u>: The alarm. A new clock with a good loud ring. Must be everybody's off today. No lights on.

To the mess hall through the mud… Across the construction site… Down the bank, jump the soft area… don't jump far enough and sink beyond my ankles. Hold my breath past the sewer.

<u>Breakfast</u>: These days, there is juice. No matter what that fellow does to the "eggs," and regardless of the excuse offered as toast, there's juice. The mess hall is steamy hot, of course.

<u>At work</u>: The ward is cool. "Wham" and one of the fellows starts half out of bed. "Oh no!" There follows a repetition of the explosion, only close enough to shake the walls this time. It goes on every minute or so for about a half hour. The patients calm with the knowledge that it's "only a bombing."

"Yeh, but whatever they're bombing, Charlie's out there. They don't just drop bombs for the fun of it."

The corpsman calls out that you can see the bombing from the door. Rose takes a look:

"Well, I've seen my first bombing… the planes go straight up afterward"… (no one comments).

<u>The routine gets underway</u>: Rounds, joking, looking, asking, telling… Orienting a new Dr.

"These fellows are what's known as the small stuff" (those with soft tissue wounds). "The VSI's (very seriously injured) go to Ward 3."

I nearly comment, but instead, replace some dressings. Dr. W means nothing personal by this. We have neither the staff, equipment, nor location to care for the seriously wounded. I know it, and these fellows already need more than we are sometimes able or inclined to give.

<u>Dr. N makes rounds</u>: He's in a good mood. Others join him. Dr. B returns with some baby clothes his wife has sent for Tommy and a recently acquired female child.

<u>The work is essentially finished by 1000</u>: "This could be one of those days"… Rose matches her tone with her posture. "Not even anyone to surgery."

I leave to check the Vietnamese tailor shop at the 616th Clearing Station for some long-ordered Bermuda's. Flares still light the area of the strike.

"You leaving us already, Captain?"

"Yep, I just had to come in to make sure everything was shaped up (smile)."

<u>1200</u>: Back on the ward, the day is indeed quiet. Rose goes to quarters for the afternoon. There's just enough for one person to do. I pass the meds.

"Is that tomato juice? Oh, okay, as long as it's not tomato juice."

"It's not tomato juice? I'd like water then."

"Hey, this guy said he'd take that shot for me."

<u>1500</u>: Inter shift report:

"Did you want a urine on Tommy? He just sat on the bag and squished it all over the bed."

<u>1600</u>: Nurses' Meeting: I am questioned about how I've set up the ward to provide a treatment room (it's not like other wards). I volunteer to immediately go to make the ward compliant (with a bit of urgency) but am assured that I should remain in the meeting. I insist, maybe even bordering on sarcasm, but things then proceed quietly.

<u>Later</u>: a cup of coffee. In Pat's area listening to tapes.

"Hello, how are you?"

"Good!"

"Liar."

"No, really", as I ease past Mac, finish the coffee and leave to rid my area of the infamous Vietnamese dresser.

A couple troops appear outside.

"You aren't throwing that out!"

"Yes, (pause) would you like it? I just got tired of it is all."

"Hey, Ed. Our first piece of furniture!"

Much laughter from others who have gathered as the dresser is carried off over the chest of a young Spec 4.

<u>Reading</u>: "Your Men at War."

Descriptions of combat and emotions surrounding such are disturbing. I glance at my helmet with the bars; it really is an honor to "'own" that. I put the book down. It's thought-provoking—too much so. We really have a soft life. Imagine watching one's friends getting shot… shot oneself.

Imagine…

**04 May 67**   <u>1800</u>: It was a good night to write a description of a routine day in VN.

**05 May 67**   Two boys and their friends, the friends being 2 large black bugs.

"Hey, Captain, look!"

To the nearest boy, "You like him?"

"Oh yes!"

"He's a nice bug?"

"Yes! He's called gif g-i-f."

"What does the bug eat?"

"That!" (As he points to the wood of the building nearby.)

They laugh uproariously and depart, each with his "gif" held affectionately on exhibit.

I think of the boy of a friend who never failed to enliven daily events with his assorted "friends". It is a good thought. I smile to myself and return to the ward.

**06 May 67** Yesterday, a patient returned to tell us how much we had done for him. After about 5 minutes, I placed him, one of about 30 men received in a period of a few hours approximately 5 weeks ago. The puzzling point was that we evac'ed 25 of those men to 3$^{rd}$ Field within 12 hours after their arrival on the ward. This individual had been shot through the left cheek, the bullet lodging in the soft palate. His face was grossly swollen when I approached him that AM. He was most uncomfortable but stable.

During rounds, he was even more anxious; I asked him what was going on with him. With difficulty, he insisted, "Ma'am, I gotta take a piss!" (Smiling to myself, I replied that the corpsman would get him a urinal!)

Yesterday, he spoke on and on about when he had been in the field. (He's since been assigned to work in the base camp where "… the only good thing about it is you're not getting shot at.") He said he was the last to get hit in an original group of 14 arriving 10 months ago. He's Puerto Rican, from Connecticut via New York City, where his father decided "to move after some guys tried to drown me. The ol' man just up and left. He come back in about a week, and we leave New York and never go back. My one brother is in his first year at Notre Dame."

He spoke of going home after leaving VN, of resigning from the Army and going back to school. ("I only have one year of college.") He spoke of the only man under his supervision that he had lost. "He disobey. The last thing I tell him before I leave was to stay down. He didn't. He disobey… they pick me up, and there is one in bag. I look…"

Later:

Lest the flavor of the land be lost… I entered the latrine of the Air Force Base in Bien Hoa tonight: Two female VN employees were there. One squatted with her back exposed. The other knelt over her, inflicting a welt about 1 inch wide the length of her vertebral column. In explanation, "She sick."

"But what about Dr.?"

A look of incomprehension…

"Doctor… this (indicating the caduceus on my collar)." She shakes her head.

"Is that good?"

"Yes, good. She sick."

And they continue, one scraping the flesh from the back of the other with the handle of a mess hall spoon.

**16 May 67** 81 days until leave.

**19 May 67** Decided I'd best not mail the last 5 pages of a letter to Warren. Sometimes one can get carried away. At any rate, it is a fairly lucid expression of feeling, and I'd rather not toss it out.

> They burned the flag of the greatest country in the world. They slapped the face of 440,000 very young men who want nothing <u>less</u> than to be in Tay Ninh, or on Hill 881, but who get up and go every time they're told to. They turned their backs on the millions of people (many of them orphans, literally starving) we are trying to help to help themselves. This is not a good war, none could be, for both sides have those groups of "young men;" it is ugly and not consistent with a neat suburban existence. I fail to understand, however, how people could not believe that Red China would not swallow this place (including Ho Chi Minh) very shortly after we left. Do they not give one damn about Tommy (Taum), aged 4 years, weight 14 pounds... for Det Sung CIDG (Civilian Defense Group) whose entire right chest the VC blew out?… for the young men who were killed less than an hour after arriving here in Vietnam (at Bien Hoa) the other night? Do they actually believe their cozy intellectual existence will survive by simply turning their backs? Have they no guts to face the unpleasant fact that the strong inherit the grief of the weak and are morally bound to give aid, while at the same time ensuring their own continued strength? Can they burn the flag that so many are dying for and not question their behavior?

> I am glad I came here, Warren. I hate it, as so many do, but we are doing the best we know how to do and, at times, doing a mighty good job. It gradually provides some answers to the

puzzling newspaper articles. It is giving help where help is needed, and (selfishly) it deepens and broadens one view of life.

Best I close, for I could not really say all or precisely what I feel tonight. No one asks that people who are not here mope around, dwelling on VN; it is only asked that they work toward giving a better way of life rather than rending that which exists. Perhaps it is they who would make the better fighters. Most of these kids don't care much for fighting—really.

Love, Mrs. Smith

**19 May 67 (continued)**  2350 PM …one way to keep one's sheets clean is not to use them! Last evening, having awakened to total darkness, it was not difficult to discern that we were having the rumored alert (only everyone had gone to the bunker while I slept on).

Shortly, I joined them and waited for Group to call it off. "We're expecting an air attack at about 2200, and we might as well be ready." (From the Chief Nurse.) Well, my heart leapt into a staccato beat before I even realized that the VC and NVN (North Vietnamese) have essentially no Air Force… then it leapt again with the thought that all sorts of things come from "the air" in a broad sense, including mortars.

We were advised to get into uniform, which we did and then returned to the bunker. 2200 came and went. Except for 12 artillery firings and a number of flares, all was quiet. We went outside and waited. Several of us chose to lie down near the quarters. It was pleasant there on Mac's poncho (though the ground consisted of an inordinate number of pebbles).

At 2330, we returned to quarters but were told to remain dressed (hence no use of sheets). The Chief Nurse further noted, "We don't know where they are." The alert was still on this morning, so the mess hall staff couldn't start breakfast until 0600. The patients ate 1 ½ hours late, but it was good to slow things down. It emphasizes the absurdity,

I think, of awakening people at that hour so they can receive trays or hustle off to the mess hall to eat.

The day was very busy, and the corpsmen quite tired. They had been up all night walking the perimeter, but they worked like beavers. We finished by 1530, and a couple more patients came in then. More transfers all day from assorted hospitals. It's a good thing Japan can't transfer back here to us.

**24 May 67**   In many respects, things are becoming rather pleasant of late. Not so long ago, Mac and I went on at great length... about what luxury is:

- having juice for breakfast
- having doors on the latrine
- a hot shower
- preparing one's own meal
- having flush johns
- a private area with a door and lock

Many of these things have been obtained. That evening a few months ago, they seemed far away though the entire round was more one of nostalgia than actual longing.

At present, there is juice for breakfast, there is sugar that pours, and latrines with doors. There are johns that flush, and private living areas. There is even a kitchen and lounge with an electric stove, and last week a literal feast of eggs, bacon, chocolate milk, bread and margarine!

**25 May 67** My order from Sears has arrived! It seems a fine thing to have replaced the poncho liner with a fitted gold corduroy bedspread and added four scatter pillows of red, gold, green and blue. It seemed equally fine to discard the faithful cardboard box and replace it with a wicker waste basket. It will all be set off smartly by installing a ceiling over my area and covering the screening with curtains.

The paint job still looks fresh, and with the rains, the dust is at a minimum. The PX (post exchange) obtained a supply of pre-recorded tapes, and I found a darkroom at Train Compound (Bien Hoa). It's no longer necessary to await leave in Japan or R&R (rest and relaxation) in Thailand to provide for some entertainment. Since the alert last week (Thurs), we have not been allowed "out of the gate," but I have not really minded terribly.

PAUL

He likes jellybeans and jumping out of airplanes. He was with the 5th Special Forces until his career was abruptly halted by shell fragments that pierced his left eye and right anterior chest wall. He'll go home now, and he's plenty happy about that. He's not so very different from precisely 1599 others who have been patients here... in many respects. He looks younger than his age of 21.

**30 May 67** The Sacred Triage (pre-op, OR, post-op)

How jealously guarded; how easily violated! Why the bluntness and emotionalism in response to thoughts such as follows?

"You know when Major M. leaves, Tam could take over post-op (They'd need a major), and maybe I could move to pre-op. Jeanne's perfectly capable of handling '4.'"

Pat replies, "She won't move!"

(or)

"With the workload as heavy as it is on (post-op), the other wards could do quite a bit to relieve it. They wanted to send us a trach patient this AM, but we couldn't take him. We don't have a suction. I think the nursing office should take a look at distribution of equipment. It could relieve a vicious cycle."

Pat, "There isn't any equipment. OR has three suction machines. Post-op's sharing a machine between every 2 people now."

"It's not ideal, but people sharing a machine? They run people through the IPPB, breathing in and out all over the same tubing."

84

Pat, "You'd know what was so bad if you ever saw one of those guys choke to death!" She responded suddenly and strongly.

"Cut the crap, Pat! We've all seen people die."

I felt much resentment at what appeared to me as a sudden leap from the question of good care to a life and death matter. Just who was suggesting that people's lives should be endangered anyway? This group of staff speak of their vast workload (from the occasional comment to the habitual griper) but don't let someone even suggest a means of lightening same, or even inquire into a means of accomplishing this. It strikes me that they need this overwork, this drama, this type of dependence from another human, far too much... and I'm sicker than hell of their "mightier than thou" responses to situations referring to who works harder, "sees" more, etc. It is reminiscent of the discussions I've heard between the infantry and armor, old troops and new, as to who witnesses more horror. Really, Ladies and Gentlemen, there's plenty of horror for everyone... as well as plenty of discomfort and indignity.

Spending one's bedtime dodging and killing "airborne" bugs 1 ½ to 2 ½ inches long is indignity enough for me, as is shaking these creatures out of one's clothing in the AM.

What the hell, they just started in again... killed one with the handy, dandy insecticide we have (Aerosol, Synergized Pyrethrin Type Il). They appear unharmed at the instant they're sprayed but shortly start convulsing and, within about 15 minutes, cease visible movement. Lovely. Their size permits an exacting study of the entire process.

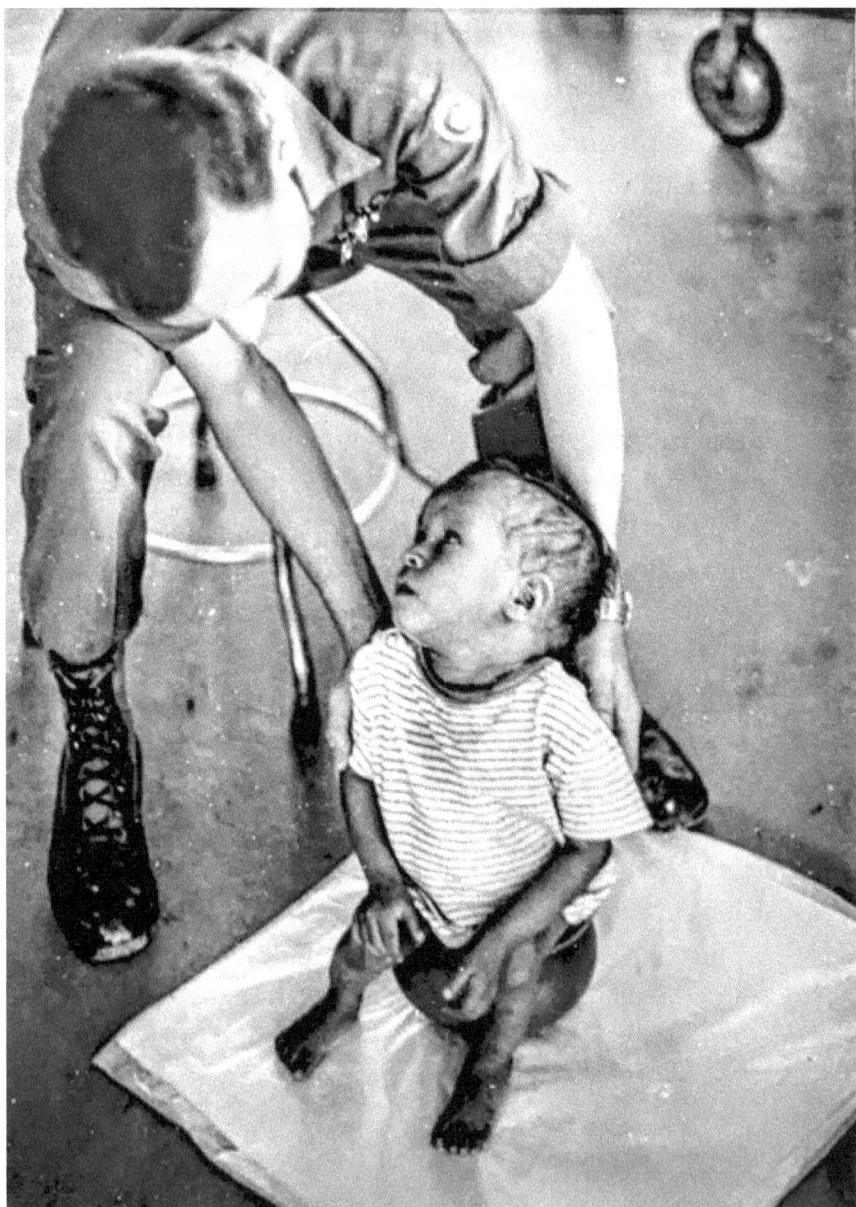

Taum on Potty

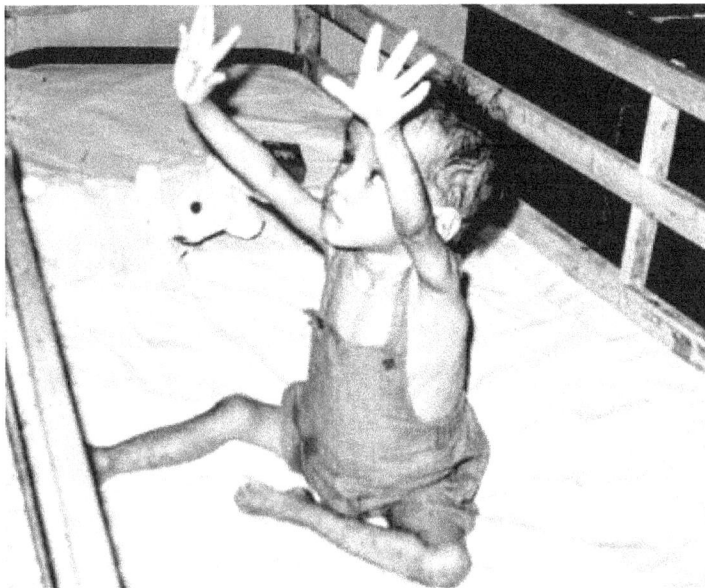

Taum on Reaching Up

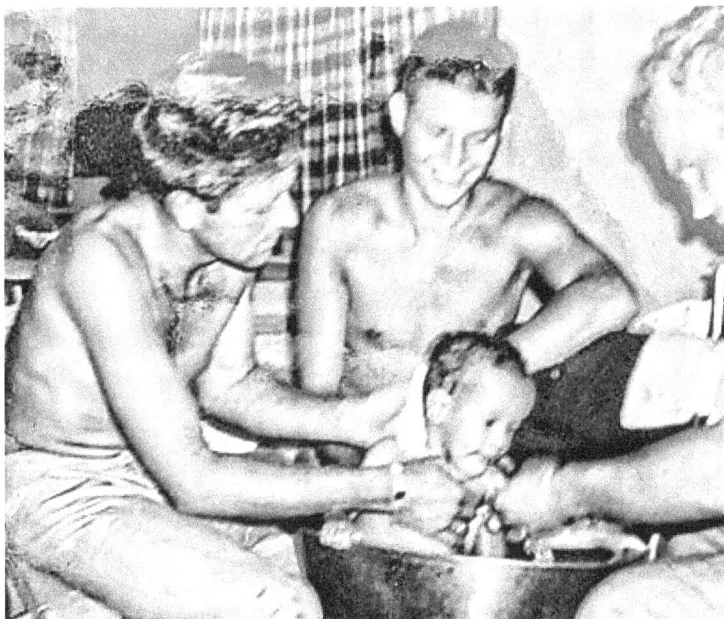

GIs bathing Taum

Fay Ferington

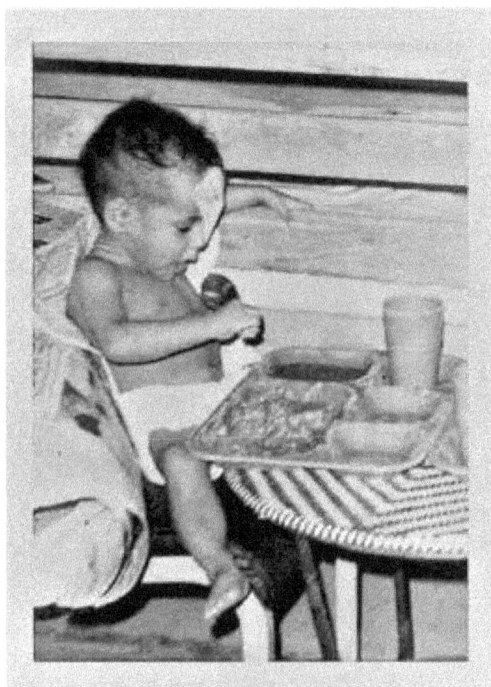

**Taum Eating**

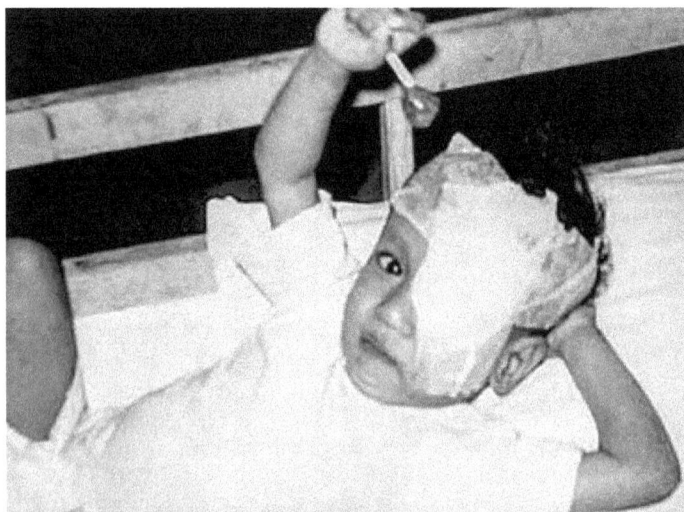

**Taum with Sucker**

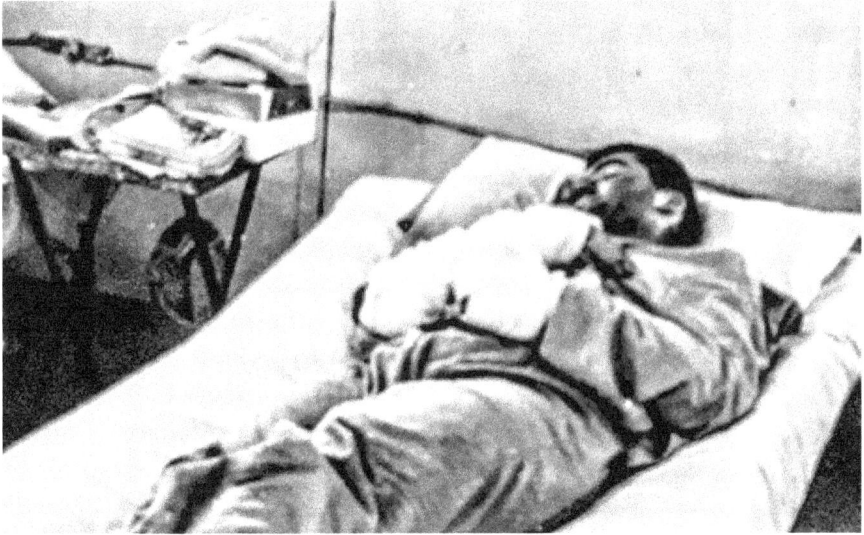

**GI with Burns**

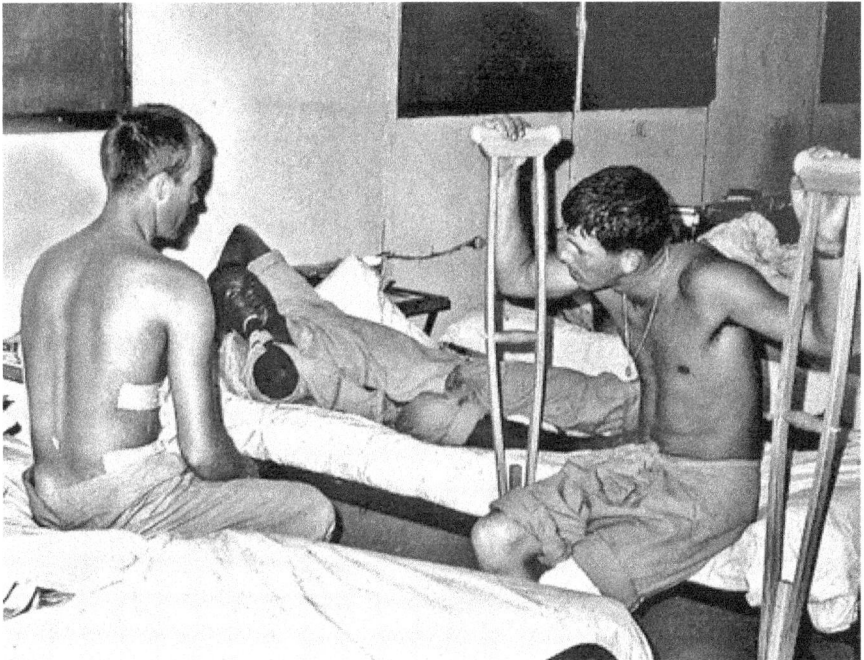

**To Return to the Field**

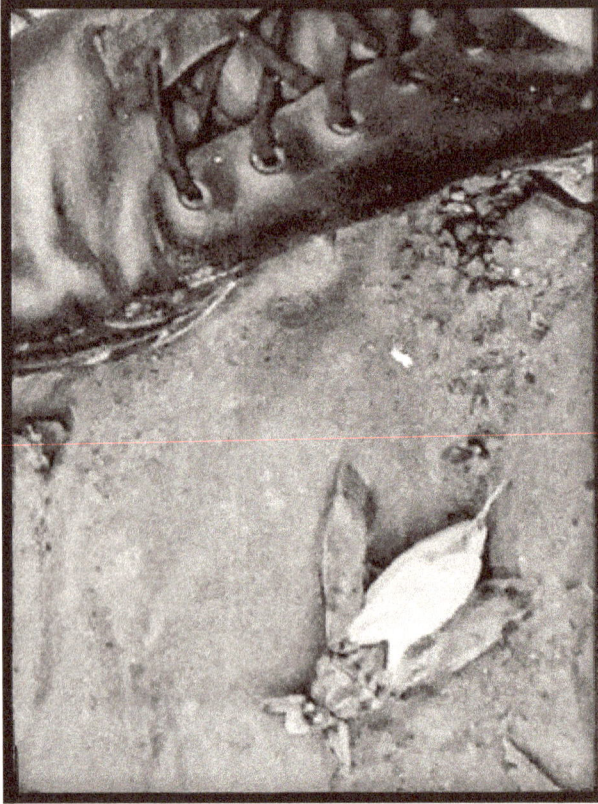

One of Many

# Chapter 8: Reflections
# (31 May 67 – 07 Jul 67)

**31 May 67** Gave a unit of blood today. Didn't see the fellow who received it, but saw his litter… "One leg gone, probably lose the other one, as well as half of his face." He stepped on a mine, so it seems. I wanted to do something rather badly when walking past the litter—or else retreat rather thoroughly.

Another patient went bad on the ward today (Strowder). That makes three in the last 1½ weeks, and I can just see another coming up. It seems a bit unusual. Though we're getting sicker patients lately, it seems more are "getting away" from these men than "got away" from Dr. Williams. We'll see, I suppose.

A pre-recorded tape is blaring: "Come on baby, let the good times roll…" The lounge is otherwise quiet. One girl sleeps; I'm reading. One leans forward intently about 6 inches from the speaker. Three others sit, apparently listening. Nobody is really moving. Their faces are thoughtful.

In *Pace Magazine,* an article contains/concentrates on "Man and His Future." A letter to the editor from a "GI in Vietnam" speaks of feelings about the loss of a friend. The music changes... "My prayer..." tears spring from some unrecognized place, and I am relieved that Bev flicks the rapid forward lever.

Judy and Phyllis enter.

"The bugs aren't really bad tonight." (Judy is frightened of bugs.)

"Last night, they were all over the place. The corpsmen thought it was funny until I started to cry. Some people are afraid of lightning. With me, it's bugs." She laughs. Someone contests Judy's statement of self-reassurance. A new topic—bugs, how large, how many, how to kill…

The hot chocolate is boiling. If it was sterile from the can, it's really sterile now. A cup of hot chocolate and a peanut stick, a good magazine… a bloody litter, a young sergeant whose abdominal wall is sloughing off. I want to cry.

**05 Jun 67**   Hard to imagine where these last five days have gone. It was a little difficult to make it through til Saturday. Knowing that it would be, I scheduled myself off on Sunday also and have slept long hours these past two days. It's had its desired effect, though, and I feel rather rested tonight.

When spending 95% of one's time between two buildings and attempting to record pertinent aspects of that period of time, it's not difficult to become rather narrow in one's viewpoint: was there juice for breakfast, were we busy on the floor, what's new at the PX, any letters at mail call, did it rain? Over and over eight months of it.

Any news is often unpleasant. In Bien Hoa, 14 deaths so far—whoever heard of a cholera epidemic in the mid-20th Century? Spec Davis, the lad who worked in the PX went on R&R and died two days after arriving in Hawaii. He had been one with whom it was possible to joke. At least he didn't die <u>here.</u>

We had some incoming mortars a couple times last week. They tended to rattle the place a bit. The shower was warm, and it was tempting to stay there and use every drop. That must be the second time that's happened around here this year.

**09 Jun 67**   Is it possible to say something of meaning for another? Is it not more probable that one will spew forth so much drivel and call it prose—or much worse—poetry?

It is raining, as it has been off and on all day. The water descends with a fierceness wholly unrelated to the familiar rains of Spring. It pelts crevices in the packed earth, it pools in depressed areas, it overflows the margins of each, and in a frenzy, tears wide the sides of drainage ditches. It comes abruptly and stops in like manner… It is as though to say, "I control me. I bridle this ferocity at will."

**12 Jun 67**  Tommy had surgery on his eyes today.

**13 Jun 67**  I signed the final draft of my RA (Regular Army) Application… "a decided asset to the RA Nurse Corps… etc."

The above is for the eyes of "need to know" people only (and I'm one of those people). It was reassuring to receive some type of evaluation after nearly 10 months in a new endeavor. The die is cast, as the saying goes—a commitment that will lead heaven knows where.

PS: I received curtains and sockets for the wall locker today—put the curtains up. They are simply elegant and the next to the final step in "home decorating" Project #1.

**15 Jun 67**  Sgt S left via air-evac yesterday. Of course, the best part of it all was seeing him leave after having seen him give up a couple weeks ago ("I think I'm going to retire right here.") He didn't die here; in fact, he isn't going to die. I carried his belongings out to the bus, and as they were lifting him aboard, he reached out his left hand and, with a wink, "It's the only way I can say thanks, Captain."

"Take care, buddy" (before thinking of the phraseology).

I thought my reaction to scenes such as these had long since subsided, but tears filled my eyes, making the brilliant sun less intense… as he left our ward with a "damn" for his recent apparent fate.

**20 Jun 67**  There must be a way to write out feelings.

**17 Jun 67** Item #1, …82 casualties to the 93rd, an almost unheard-of number all at once. One sleeps, oblivious to the gathering chaos or one rushes to duty, with the certainty of his or her usefulness... or one waits, refraining from a drink lest by some unlikely probability, one's services are needed to help with the paperwork or to run errands… It is possible to maintain a waiting posture for a goodly period of time.

It is possible to contain one's outrage throughout with reasonable humor. It is not dissimilar, however, to the dilemma of being caught in barbed wire: Do not move to the left where the barb of being unneeded lies waiting. Do not move to the right, where you might affect your consciousness with the depressive effect of alcohol. Remain alert, that having seen pain and quantities of blood on occasion—that having seen the violence of weaponry on occasion, you might realize the unspeakable tragedy adjacent to that awareness. Do not partake, and do not refuse to if asked. Remain aware. Do not curse the idleness of your evening—offer solace to the players in the "drama." Give care to the helpers and you have helped.

**18 Jun 67** Item #2, …42 casualties to the 93rd. Be aware, do not shrink from an account of leaches crawling in open wounds—from the knowledge that the wounded, dirty, crying soldier is 19 years old and that our own artillery did this. Do not dwell on a vision of the rice paddy from whence he was lifted—you have not earned that right.

Evacuate the patients, remake the beds, arrange the bulletin board according to SOP, give a class on the fire plan, on the alert procedure, write an efficiency report or a recommendation for an award…

**27 Jun 67** I believe there is good and there is evil. I believe human beings are good. I believe love to be the greatest good and deception the essence of evil, in any form. I believe:

1. It is neither to the individual's credit nor discredit be he of greater or lesser natural endowment.
2. It is the individual's responsibility to development, that endowment to its utmost limit and apply it in as beneficial manner as possible.

3. If there were absolutes of dependence and independence, it would be more admirable to be independent.

4. An individual must love himself.

5. It is the responsibility of the strong to assist those weaker. It is immoral to use that strength against the weaker.

6. Under given circumstances, an act ordinarily considered wrong is necessary.

7. There are some ideas of such pure intent that they cannot be defiled by the ineptness of those who seek to apply them. Nursing, as a form of service, is one of those ideas.

8. Life is basically a tragic process.

9. As was recently written in *Pace Magazine*, quoting Victor Frankl: Happiness is achieved most readily while least actively seeking such.

10. Retaliation in any form is most often wrong, as the absence of defense is stupid.

11. If one is fully aware of the sacrifice required to attain a given goal, one should weigh this price and bare it without regret in pursuit of that goal.

12. A person's endowments are vastly tempered by his early environment, but at one decisive point, he must recognize himself as the primary source of influence and declare: "…from now on, with what I have, I will make me."

13. In order to live most meaningfully, an individual must be willing to entertain given risks. The depth of the experience demands that he be aware of these risks.

14. A "big" human being will take (or receive) comfortably that which another needs to give if such is consistent with his value system. He will refuse with equal comfort if such is not the case.

**03 Jul 67** Tommy went "home" last Friday (30 June). His eyes were straightened to the point where he could use each of them to obtain a 3rd dimension. His skin was completely healed, but he never gained beyond 20 pounds. Something in the little fellow resisted all our fine medical might—in the final analysis. In addition to this, he never really walked. On the positive side, his original total lethargy disappeared. He played and smiled and poked into every corner of the ward that he could get to as though possessed by some benevolent spirit of inquiry. He stood and leaned against one and gazed softly upward. One would guess that he no longer expected only pain from his environment.

As a child, it seemed difficult to await Christmas Day. How many of those Christmases will reappear upon touching down at Travis AFB. One will leave the Base and return to the stream of everyday events in San Francisco, or LA, or NYC or in a small rural community somewhere in between. One will walk with others as though one had never left one's homeland and recall this year with an apathy, an anger, or a sorrow, alluding the descriptive power of words. One will avoid detail, and some will read depth into that avoidance. Will they know the depth of accepting the unacceptable?

**07 Jul 67** Jeanne told me she had a tape, "Angels in Fatigues," a salute to the ANC (Army Nurse Corps) by the 1st Infantry Division. Having just played it, some comment is necessary:

I cannot buy it. The smiling wounded soldier; angelic nurse; the effective MedCap (Medical Civil Action Program); the melodramatic glory. In the first place, the 93rd is not in a jungle and not now in a small clearing. The 93rd, along with what are probably, by now, thousands of other unpainted, clapboard buildings, is located on Route 1 in the now treeless, grassless, rain-drenched/dust bowl of Long Binh Post. It presently has paved roads, central electricity (as of yesterday), and since December, a passable OC (Officer's Club). We don't perform miracles; in the short run, only some are summoned in mass casualties, and we are hardly angels.

The newly wounded don't smile a good deal, nor have I seen many nurses clasping hands or writing letters except as sometimes provided for those who are dying. Most are too busy changing bloody dressings, soaking infected wounds or completing a myriad of other tasks (even making sure that the beds are lined up for weekly inspection). Taking patients to Ton San Nhut for evacuation is considered a foul task by many, meaning spending hours organizing transportation and supervising the loading of litters. Nurses are probably working harder in Japan and the States than some of us and receiving less pay for each.

The tape just doesn't come off. There is no glamour, and as once noted, drama is very undramatic when one is in the center of it. There are VC all around us, and as one person said at lunch, "If we had to move further back, there would be no place to go but through VC territory.

## Cycle of Care:

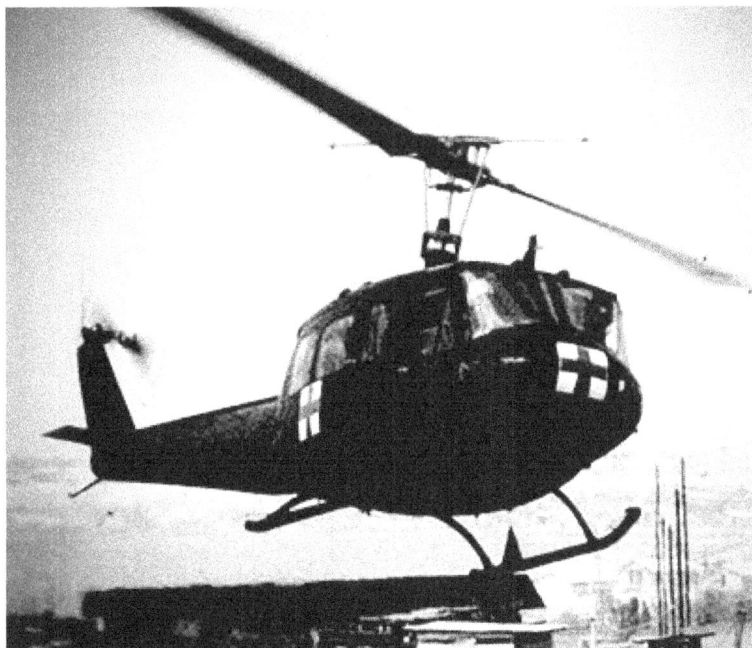

**Huey Evac Landing**

97

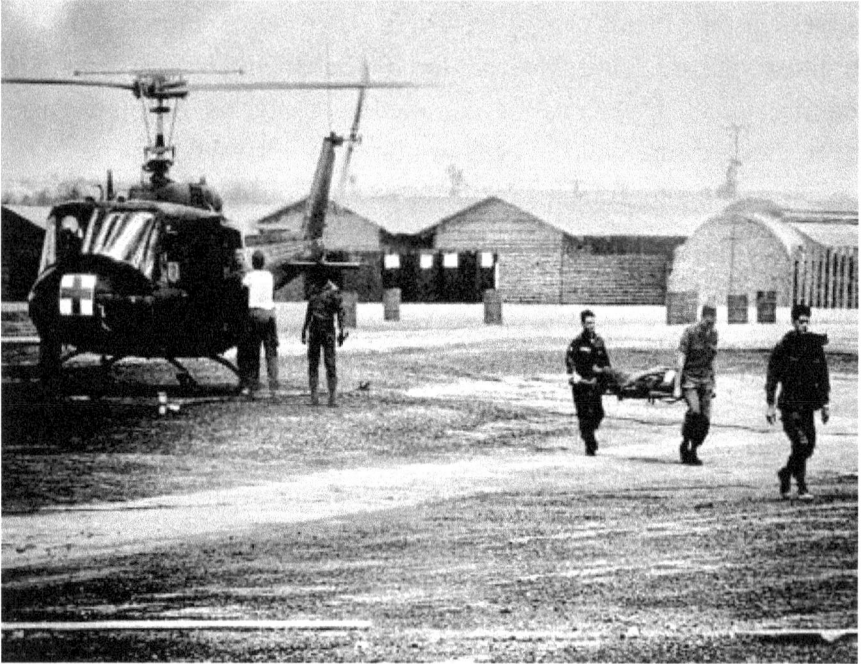

To Pre-Op

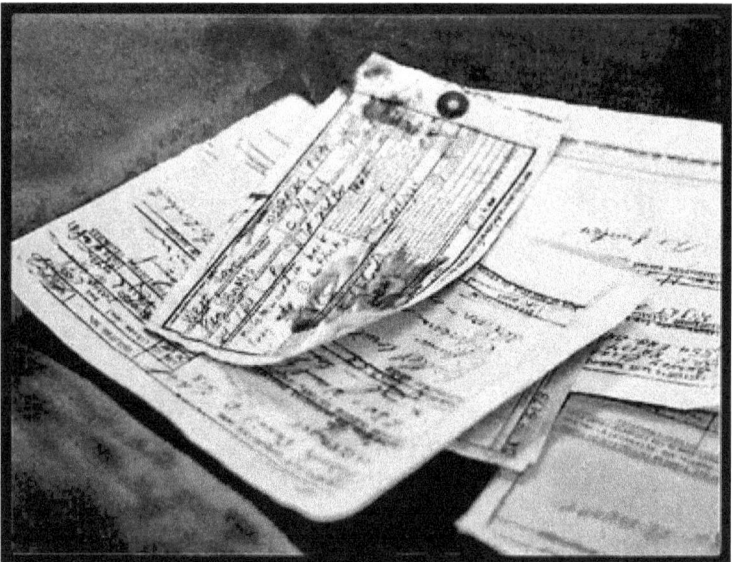

Medical Record from the Field

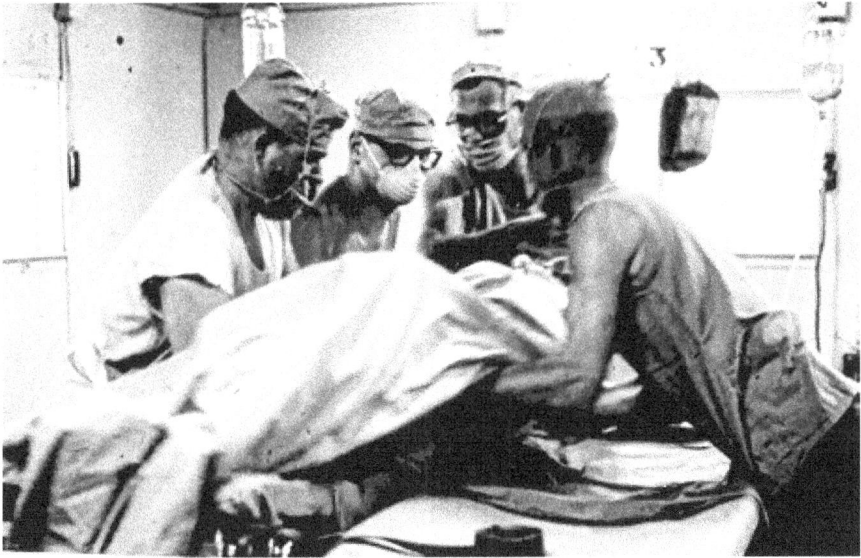

In OR

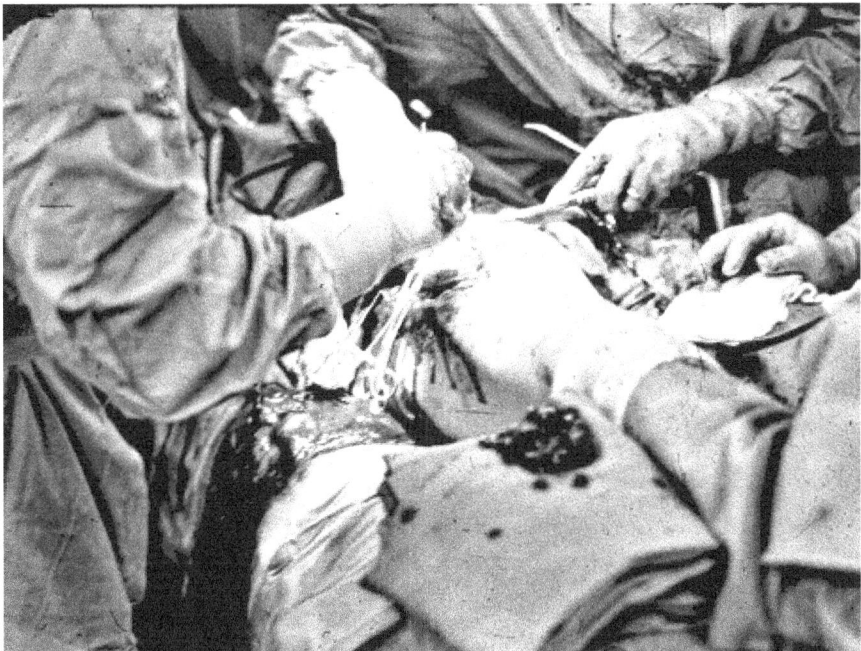

Surgery

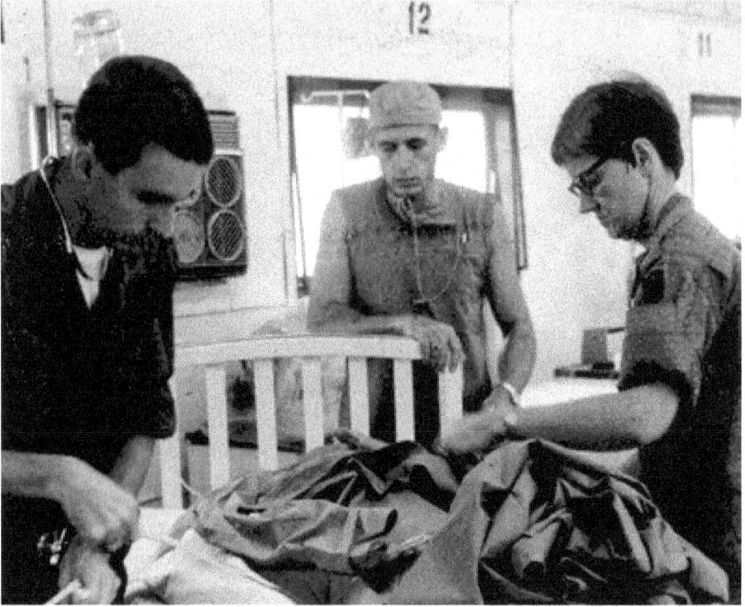

In Recovery Room

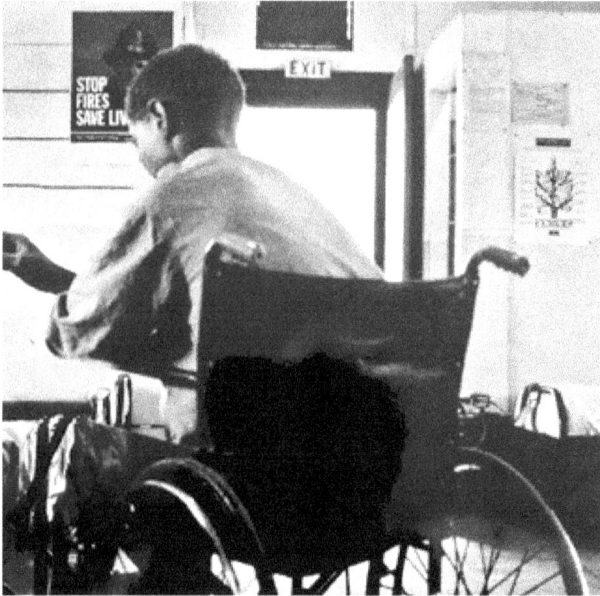

Awaiting Evac to Japan

# Chapter 9: Short-Timer
# (09 Jul 67 – 24 Aug 67)

**09 Jul 67** Last summer, precisely one year ago, I watched TV documentaries on the war in Vietnam.

Tonight, it is quiet. I sit on a straw mat, a red patterned straw mat placed over a cement floor. An identical mat is stretched just under the steel roof. A news program is broadcast from AF (Armed Forces) radio, Saigon. The above scene has been repeated so often that my mind strains to answer the question: "What had I expected our life here to be like?" I think back to when it seemed possible that people finished their tours and left Vietnam when the simple prospect of boarding a plane was not beyond one's imagination.

I guess I expected a type of adventure. I know I expected much physical discomfort in daily living conditions and a good deal of hard work. I expected an awareness of the war, and for the first few weeks, there apparently was. There were sounds and sights and smells, which were unfamiliar. There was the ever-present generator, the hum of the fans of each occupant of our quarters. There was the helicopter. (It coughs and chugs and pops as it swings low over the hospital.) There were jets. (They snarl through one's ears—they are supreme.) There was the racing of the motor of deuce-and-a-half (2 ½ ton) trucks, the clanking of tanks and APCs (armored personnel carriers) over route 1; going out and coming back, they sound the same in either direction. There was the strange nasal quality of the VN tongue. All these sounds grown familiar.

There were new sights—and new variations on old sights, all alluding to the war around us; a group of soldiers hushed, awed nearby, inquiring about a wounded friend, their weapons worn as casually as their muddy boots. There were always weapons, as a matter of fact. There were slicks (gunships), one of which once carried me to a party near Tay Ninh but never on that mission for which they were designed. There were sunsets, one once noted as being beautiful. There were shacks called homes, made of thatched weeds, or tin or cardboard, their inhabitants nearly always smiling at the visitor under their cone-shaped hats. There were more tents then… tents with the flaps tied down over mud floors or rolled back from wooden walls. There were medivac choppers and litters and dirty bandages from the field. There was a VN man coughing up a 12-inch worm as he awakened from surgery.

Strangest of all, there were smells, and it seemed they were all unpleasant. The outdoor latrine was offensive, but not nearly so much as a visit to the Bien Hoa Market, where cuts of meat hung defenseless from the flies and the continual sun. There was the "rat-man." The nature of his work made the odor worse. He went from building to building carrying his can of poison over one shoulder, spraying around and under each foundation.

On the ward, there was a mix of smells. In the PX, it was one of sweat, stale, pungent sweat soaking the back of nearly everyone's fatigues. Once, during New Year's Eve, there was the odor of gunpowder. I wonder if it smells that way in the field (probably only if one is close enough to smell Charlie's.) Sights and sounds and smells; do they make an experience?

**12 Jul 67**   I bought a stereo! The components have been assembled in the entertainment unit that was created out of the bookcase. What more satisfying sound than the crispness of the guitars, the fullness of a bass viol?

**13 Jul 67**   It was 2315. The evening had been quiet, so much so as to make the hours interminably long. Some of us had just finished work and met each other at the officers' club. It was a small space, and it was crowded with strangers. In the middle of a reasonably searching discussion on how to improve the health professions, a hearty "Hello!" as though from an old friend. A few words of superficial exchange and then, "How have you been?" from Tony.

"Fine, I hear you're living the life of Reilly now, Tony."

"Who told you that?"

"Well, aren't you in Bien Hoa now?"

He follows with a defense and an invitation to join him for a drink… then a plea to do so… and I agree.

She was over in the corner with a WO (Warrant Officer) 10 years her junior. He leaned against her—accepting her caresses. Ultimately, he moved to leave, though she moved with him in a mildly restraining gesture. His voice in an out-of-context statement above the monotone of Tony's. "You're hard-core nursing, aren't you?" Her answer is lost.

As he gazes with a half-smile, she makes her way to another group. She is very drunk. On duty, she is the keeper of the lives of the seriously wounded. On duty, she is alert, efficient, thorough; she is the giver of analgesics, the one who stops bleeding, provides aid in emergencies; she is a welcome sight. Tonight, she relieves no one's discomfort but her own. Perhaps she is "hard-core." Perhaps she is lonely.

Tony continues, "You think I'm a bad guy—have another beer. Here I am trying to tell you war stories, and you're not even listening."

"I'm sorry, Tony. Go ahead."

Talking and drinking, he speaks of being recommended for the Silver and the Bronze Star. "I don't have a degree, so I had to get a couple of medals. Should get promoted now. Hey, did you extend? I once thought if anything was worth something, it was life, but it isn't. You know where I'm going to spend leave—San Francisco!" (He says he has a wife and child in North Carolina.) "…if I can make it through a month on $1000."

He laughs, and I remember why the club is so rarely a pleasant retreat. It's very late now. He gets his beret and once more a plea, this time to walk me to quarters. Once more, an out-of-context statement… "I lost 8 men…"

**15 Jul 67** A person must need to be rather egocentric to keep a diary, particularly one such as this, consisting largely of notations of one's reflections. So many of us are at a point in life where it is as yet impossible to believe that one's life is insignificant. Surely, there must be some meaning to the abilities, the visions of significance cannot have occurred without reason... to be extinguished without an impact?

**17 Jul 67** For the second night in a row, I find it difficult to sleep. I'm excited about many things. I have tomorrow off and have not been off the compound in seven days. Barb and I will have breakfast at Bien AFB, then I believe I will take some photos (black and white). By then, the PX should be open, and perhaps they will have some records left of the hundreds they received last week—good ones too! The afternoon will be time to enjoy the cool sounds of the stereo unit.

There is a good possibility of R&R in about three weeks. Five days in Hong Kong (unless they cancel it because of the riots there)… and I believe I'll send some souvenirs home… some jewelry for mother, leather sandals or something like that for Dad, some Thai silk for Marguerite and Theta, some Chinese money for the kids. Time to take photos and get some printed and have a room in the most luxurious hotel I can afford. A chance to dress up, to eat out, to take a walk—to see people just plain living. I am also excited because, sometime in the next month, there should be orders for the States, and I then I think I'll frame them.

Lastly, there is Dian. Perhaps I will see him walk one day. He is an ARVN, hit once with an M-16 round, blowing out the head and neck of the femur, the acetabulum, and his abdominal wall after tearing his bowel and bladder to pieces. He has been hospitalized at the 93rd for the past 4 months. He will be presented at an in-service meeting this Friday. Sometimes the prospect of his recovery is so exciting that it's difficult to wait. What was a gaping abdominal wound is nearly entirely filled in with granulation tissue and, with that, the perforation of his bladder. His bowel was anastomosed, and a loop colostomy made, which he needs only minimally now. Soon the sump tube can be removed. His bed sores are healing well, and last week he was out of bed on a tilt board for the first time since his injury. If we can keep his recently rekindled interest in life sustained, if his wife will continue to visit, in short, if we can help him through these remaining weeks of discomfort when he often despairs, Dr. W says there is a chance he could develop a type of sesamoid bone in which the femur might ride, and maybe he could eventually walk. We cannot speak with words, but we speak, and his smile occurs more often now.

Somehow Dian makes me think of Phan. I will never forget what I said to him, nor will I ever know what he has done to our men. Phan was a VC. I will remember his expression of delight at coming on a picture of a 1967 Cadillac (in *Life* magazine) and then his expression of pain at losing his leg. I will remember sharing a cigarette with him and his refusal to cry. I will remember that he was too young to have a beard like the others.

**19 Jul 67**   As it turned out, I worked yesterday until 2300, helping out in the OR and supervising the Units. I awoke this AM to a sparkling sky, peaceful with its groupings of cumulus clouds.

"Last night, I dreamed there was a war. The choppers were bringing in casualties. The OR was going strong at midnight, the rain was pelting down… It must have been a dream because this AM, the ground wasn't even damp." Dave smiles at the humorless joke, and one is confident that he understands what is being said.

"That was the foulest amputation I've ever seen—probably because the bullet did most of it before he got to surgery."

Directly across from that table, Dr. W had been finishing up a hemi-hepatectomy. If the Lieutenant lives, he will be the first to survive such a procedure in Vietnam. Adjacent to him lay a young man whose hand was cut in several places, stripped of all flesh underneath. In a moment of drunken exuberance, he'd placed it in a fan.

The fourth table had been idle for several minutes. Observing the lateness of the hour, I left to make rounds. People were busy, but everything was OK.

Later today:

> Somewhere there is fighting,
> I hear explosions
> and I hear them
> cut a path through air
> as sound wave crashes
> over sound wave.
> Oblivious, the man
> whose leg came off
> (last evening)
> searches for a chance
> to have it shot
> and then come here.

## 21 Jul 67

> I listen to helicopters
> ...stereo and artillery.
> I drink beer from a can,
> I am not proud.
> I sweat and work and wait.
> (I miss my home but
> where is that?)
> I wear Bermudas
> ...made in Hong Kong
> while sitting on a sandbag
> ten rows back from Elvis Presley.
> (Until it starts to rain.)
> I tend the harvest of the war
> ...from eight to four.

**25 Jul 67**   There are times when a direct effort should be made to clarify feelings. I'll be damned if that's as easy to do as it is to say.

"You coax the blues right out of the horn—Mame."

And so, the song goes on to explain that the "whole plantation's humming" and that Mame makes the "cotton easy to pick." The song is so inherently poignant. Can the joyous yearning of this music be even remotely related to the phenomena we hear of in Detroit?

Today, rumors were abounding of the direct hit on the 3rd Surg. It was hit. None of the patients were wounded. There were 17 staff who received various fragment wounds. Despite this, I had an impulse to write and offer solace to those in Michigan; to whom?... To speak, for surely there must be forces capable of stemming the riots that have ignited the States. Oh God, can they not fathom the consequence, should the violence continue? Would it not be identical to Vietnam? Is it not now?

Frankly, I become very angry. How dare they try to turn the United States into a battleground? Stokely Carmichael, are you mad? You are leading thousands into a kind of madness. Is it that bad? Is war preferable? Are you that consumed in hatred?

I feel a childlike desire to "just tell them." Surely, if they knew... but, of course, they do know. It is those of us here, or in equally isolated areas, who, in our own world, proceed to idealize our home, to minimize its inadequacies.

**27 Jul 67**   A day slipped by nearly unnoticed. The 26th of July. At the moment, I am vastly soothed by the Chad Mitchell Trio. In addition, there was the most pleasant surprise of a homemade roast and two cups of coffee today.

The 26th of July ...it was a routine day. After work, I dropped in to see Pat and Maggie for a cup of coffee. It wasn't quite done. They talked. Marianne stopped by. She felt particularly bad. Her extension had been refused, and as a result, plans for a visit to Hawaii as well.

The lieutenant with the hemi-hepatectomy died...

**06 Aug 67**  This afternoon, I set up a uniform for R&R in Hong Kong. In 48 hours, God willing, I should be there. I look at the uniform, worn once since last 20 October, and I am proud. I feel deeply about it. The campaign ribbons—a mere two—I look at them and literally calculate 6 months each. No one, no one who has not experienced this war, can rightfully wear them, and therefore, they are precious. That person who wears them will be familiar with phrases like Operation Attleboro or Operation Junction City. He will have shared the apathy, the impulses to "break out," the hopeless realization that were there a "way out," one would choose not to take it. The only "way out" is to endure 365 days of unchanging heat and boredom (or, at times, fear). It is he alone who will truly understand how tragedy could be desired as a relief of that boredom. There have been times when I have actually wondered if the period remaining could be endured… "Only let me away from here. Let me board a plane and fly away. Let me see the United States again. Let me complete my assignment and go home."

**08 Aug 67**  I am in Hong Kong. It is interesting (to me) to note that while the prospect of theatre, music, tours, and good food was exceedingly pleasant, my response has been that of one who expected all these fine things to be waiting. It is somewhat more noteworthy that the growing feeling of confinement, experienced so recently, has faded. I was not even mindful of its passing. So much for it. I am not home, but Vietnam is a world away.

I note the uniform on my bed. I am proud to wear it. While walking through the lobby, a thought crossed my mind:

"American women are soft."

"They are not soft, see! I am an American woman, and I travel alone back to Vietnam. American women are hard as nails."

But then, I guess I'm not that representative of American womanhood—and I guess I'm not that strong either…

**09 Aug 67**  It is not difficult to fill the hours. The schedule is followed and indeed embellished by spontaneous happenings—the morning on the harbor, yielding a myriad of photos of junks and families living thereon—the afternoon frustrating at the China Fleet Club for they have little or no clothing—the evening gratifying after a lobster dinner and shortcake… after one and a half hours at a movie theatre viewing good photography and a warm human story ("A Man and a Woman").

**10 Aug 67**   Shopping from street to street… a dress, a painting… the evening listening to Schumann…

**11 Aug 67** …a beaded blouse, presents for Mother and Dad, cloth (Thai silk) for Marguerite and Theta… Later, I picked up some prints from negatives made when I was in Japan. They are better than I had a right to anticipate. They will finish my area at the 93$^{rd}$. Their content is the beauty so lacking in our day-to-day work. After dinner, I had a delightful evening of conversation with a US businessman (until 0100). We made arrangements to meet for dinner today.

Before retiring… recalling a bus tour of the new territories, the mountains, the "walled city" (with the antiquity of poverty), the freedom of just driving for three hours, it has been a good 3 days.

**14 Aug 67**   Returned from Hong Kong yesterday and spent the afternoon sleeping (and the evening listening to music.) Pat is most enthusiastic about a new record. It's by Aretha Franklin.

I checked the mail, rather expecting orders—Mac received hers. There were none. Later, I cleaned the area from stem to stern—walls, floor, the throw rug, bug net, and bedspread, and flipped the mattress—then gave everything a liberal dose of "6-12" (insecticide). Everything shines tonight, and it's a comfortable feeling. I hadn't noticed how really shabby it had begun to look.

**19 Aug 67**   I have "completed" my tour in Vietnam—only 100 days to go!

23 Aug 67 This evening, I aired the duffle bag, sprayed the trunk, and packed some uniforms. I packed all of my boxes of slides in the

carry-on Samsonite and stored it under the bed. It's the one thing I couldn't bear to lose.

**24 Aug 67** In Vietnam, there is a syndrome—the newcomer's syndrome, or more accurately, the new supervisor's syndrome. They speak to one and then continue gazing benignly as though expecting some additional comment, as though awaiting some tangible sign of one's year of experience. It is as though they are, as yet, not involved, and indeed, they are not—not yet.

They are manifestly concerned with the wounded, checking personally, encouraging—"They are so good!" It is as though they are still believers in the "myth of war"—that the boys die heroically, the girls serve courageously. I venture that if they have any strength remaining, the boys die cursing the circumstances of their death, and the girls serve uncomplainingly because to complain is to imply hope, something they have renounced long ago.

Some of the boys speak of longing for a soft tissue wound or of blowing off a foot, and some of the girls, when they do speak, wish to go home, professing a willingness to do "almost anything" to leave.

So, to the believers in the myth, I say, "No, they are not so good. They are no different than their friends at home. They have a job to do, one that offers little alternative but to do it. They will surely disappoint you one day, for one day, the apathy will recede, and the first sign of this will be the capacity to be angry that they have been set apart, that they may never return to that time before they first saw the result of war, to that time before they accepted the possibility of their own death; to that time before they were host to cockroaches, lice, parasites and an assortment of fungi."

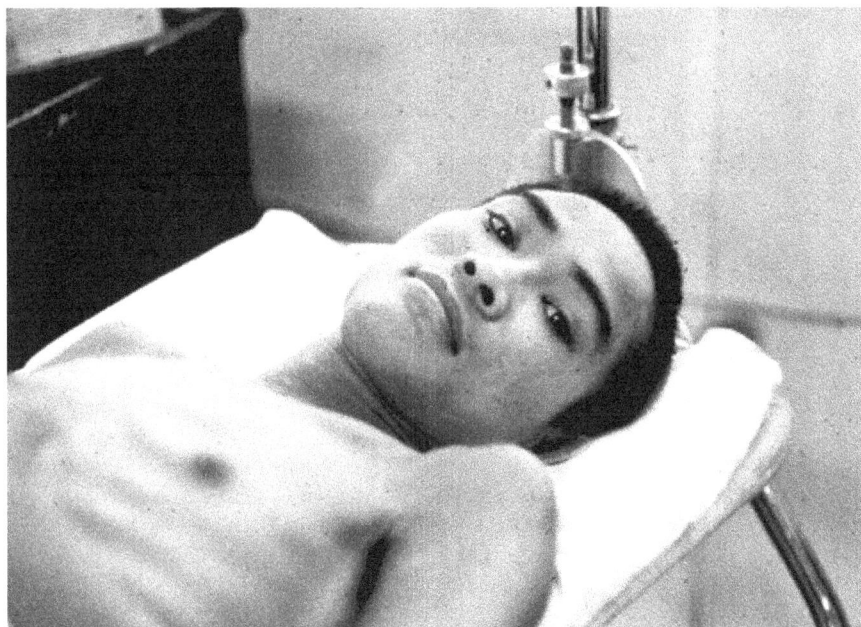

Dian

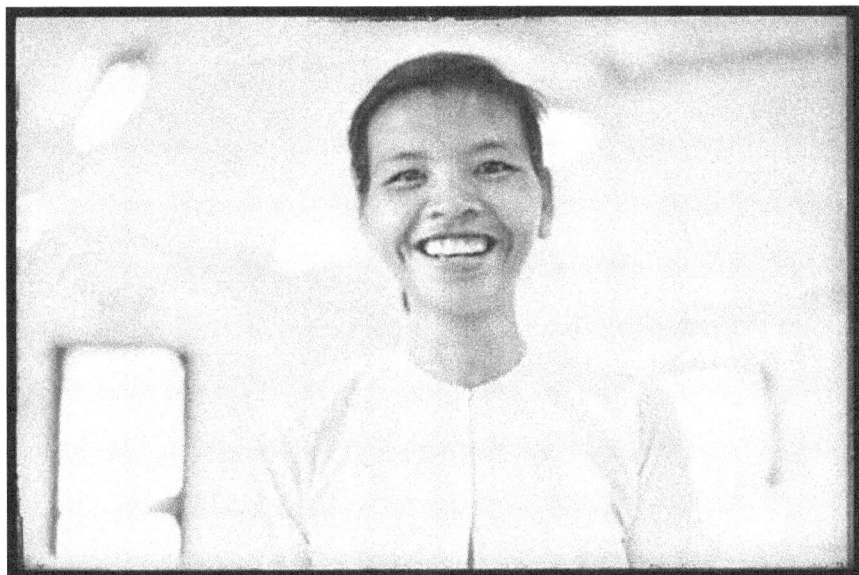

Dian's wife visited only once.

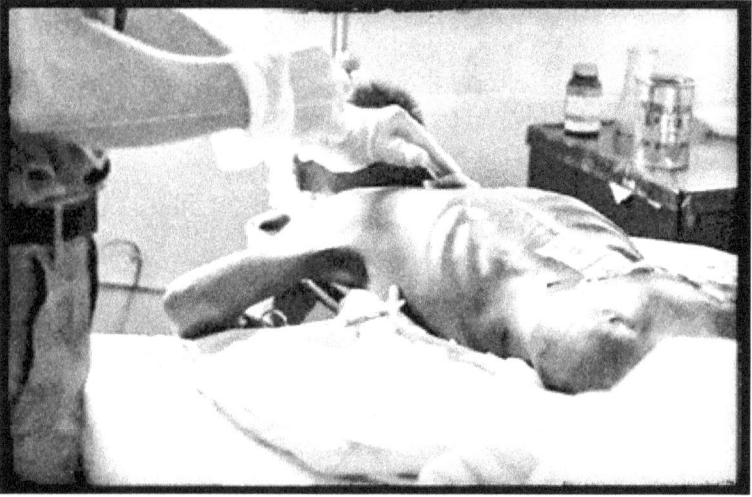

Treating Dian's skin lesions, after he began to recover from a gunshot wound to his lower back.

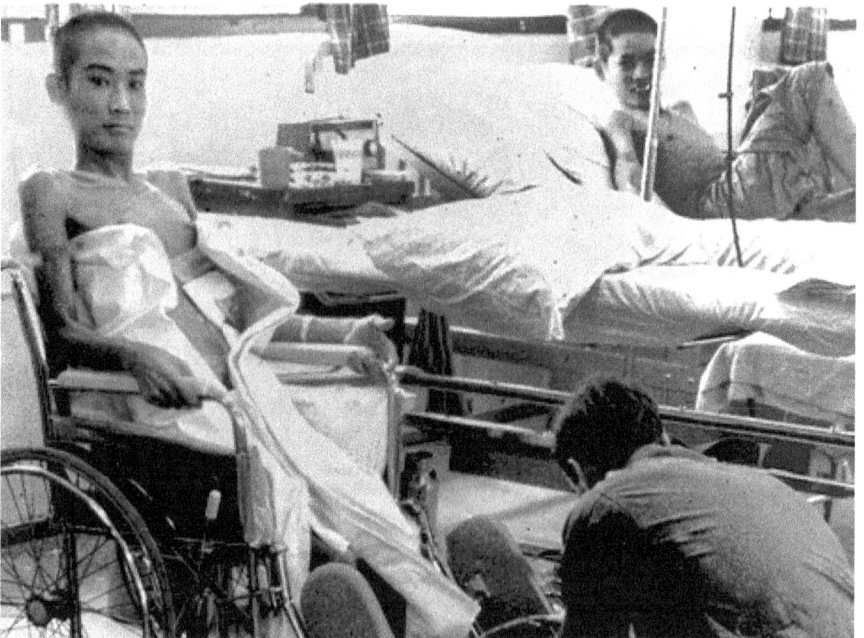

Dian Feeling Better

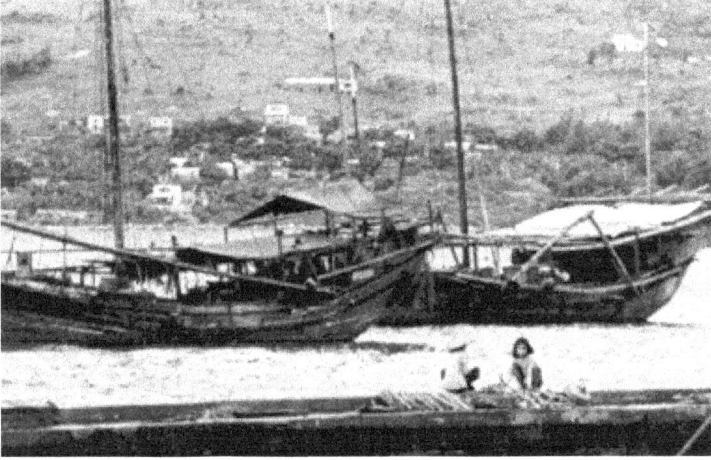

Hong Kong Harbor Scene

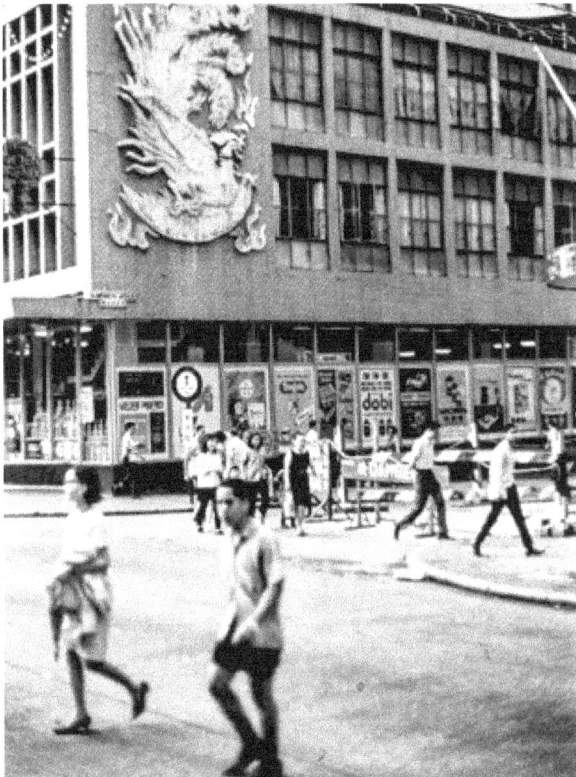

Hong Kong Street Scene

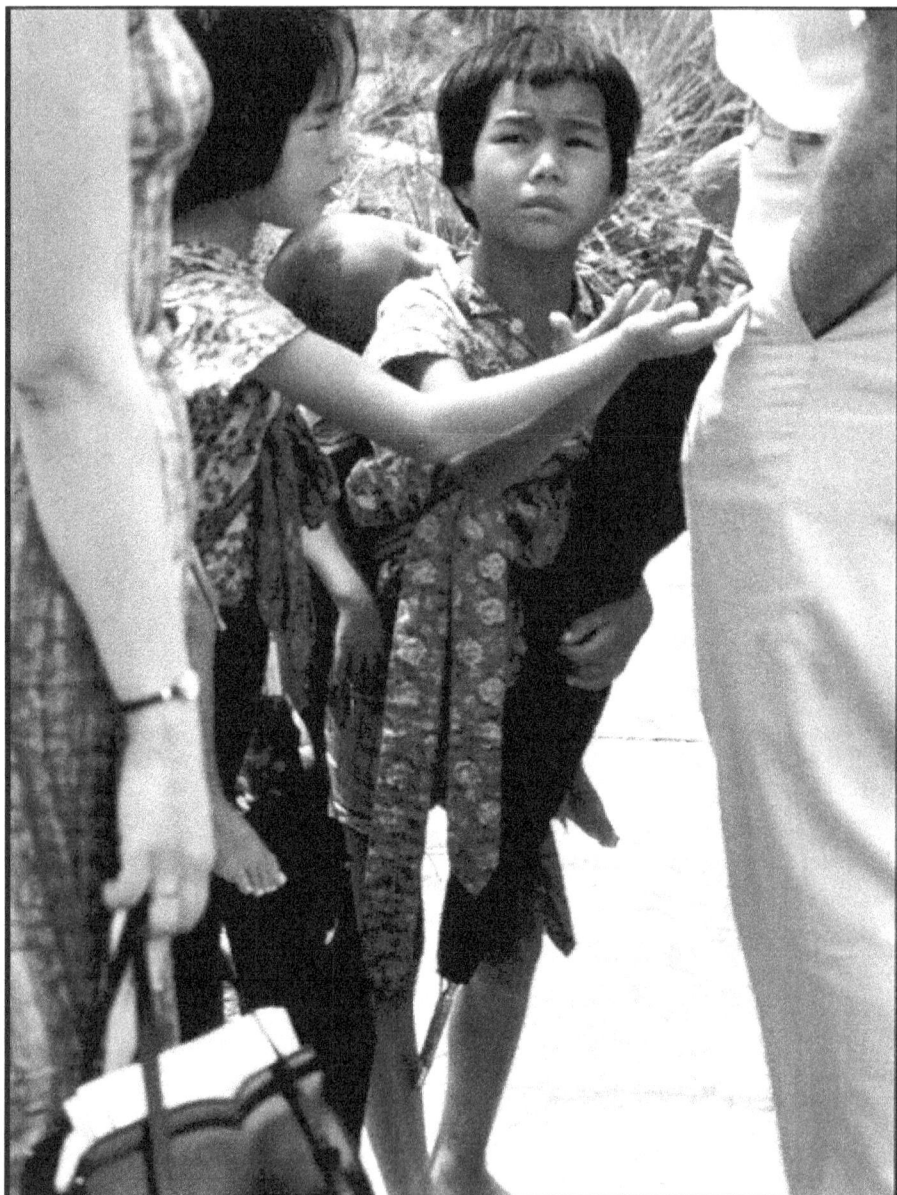

A Different Hong Kong Street Scene

# Chapter 10: Looking Toward Home (26 Aug 67 – 25 Sep 67)

**26 Aug 67** It is a Saturday evening. The kids are whooping it up next door, singing "Deck the Halls with…" I pronounce their effort foul in order to encourage greater volume (which they produce obligingly). I repeat the above in tones of marked consternation—this time from the door of Pat's area and am rewarded for this further magnanimity by a cup of coffee aimed in my general direction. Marianne joins the chaos with a recording of actual carols… and the mood changes. The carols evoke memories of assorted contexts. As I leave, I wish that she'd turn them off.

Later, Mag donned her gas mask and proceeded to appear quietly in the shadows in the hallway… quite a fright to see her standing there in that thing. I wonder if others feel as restless as I tonight. The sensible thing to do would be to go to bed.

Shirley just stopped by on her way to the 90th Replacement. She's going home tomorrow. There was very little to be said except the customary:

"If you go to Fitz (Fitzsimmons Army Medical Center, Denver), I'll see you."

"Oh, are you going to Fitz?"

"Yes, Mac and I'll be together."

"You'll be yelling at each other!"

We smile and joke briefly about the ammo dump "going up," almost wishing it would and slightly fearful that it could.

"Well, have a good flight—and get some sleep." (Shirley looks very tired.)

"I guess they're expecting something tonight."

"You heard that too?"

"Who told you?"

"I don't remember." (We've heard this type of thing so many times, and still, there is a slight apprehension. I wonder if the others have heard the rumor. No one mentions it if she has, except Shirley).

"Is Pat in? Her light's out."

"She's one of those tensor things—and a ceiling. She's in, really."

"OK, well, take care."

"Yes, I shall."

**27 Aug 67** Rather like doing pushups (or pullups or whatever one does). Twenty-five; Twenty-s-i-x; T-W-E-N-T-Y-S-E-V-E-N…

George is a patient, one of those unfortunate souls whose perception of the world is so bleak that he must verify his sensual intake by acts ensuring bleak responses. He recognizes my threat to befriend him and proceeds with thrusts such as:

"You don't have one thing to complain about, you rear echelon people." (At my remark about coming to work in a poncho and leaving in same.)

"I…"

"You volunteered, so don't gripe!"

"Yes, I…"

"You flunkies!"

"What is your grade soldier?" (Only half concealing my growing irritation, seeking to address him as Pfc of Spec…)

"E-2 Sir! Ma'am! You want to bust me, go right ahead!"

"Oh George, damn it, shut up for a minute." (With decreasing irritation and a growing note of patience.)

"I can't do that, ma'am. You might win if I'm quiet."

"Win what, George?"

For the first time, he remains quiet. Eventually, I tell him that I did indeed volunteer and am happy that I did, but this is not true for all nurses in RVN; some are even separated from spouses like many of the men are.

"Yeh, but we're doing a job while you flunkies back here…"

I let it drop and leave the ward, thinking that he (George) is an example of how the most unpleasant of reputations can be attributed to the GI, and it occurs to me that George might be the most frightened of the lot, were we ever hit. He'd probably be as demanding of sustenance as a child… Undoubtedly, I found that thought comforting at George's expense. I ponder the infection in his foot that brought him here and dismiss the incident in favor of the pleasant prospect of a soda.

**29 Aug 67** At times, I can only feel blessed. I remember, as a child, turning from my mother's attempt to tell me this, defending myself from her love. I remember the acute embarrassment. And now, 20 years later and 10,000 miles away, her words and their meaning are felt most vividly. For it is in this relative and lasting isolation that I have survived. The religious would say God grants strength. Indeed, and perhaps in no more profound manner than by means of our endowments at birth; our varying capacities to perceive.

I recall first seeing a mountain. It was in Southern Arizona across miles of desert, beyond the clouds, it seemed. It was ragged, a luminous pink despite the haze. I recall a grey rainy day gazing at the Atlantic Ocean, attempting to grasp a conception of its seemingly endless horizon. I recall the delight of the winter's first snow, the green of spring leaves and the listless days of a NY summer. I can feel this, and I can nurture such awareness.

I am able to rest as a result of clarifying confusing responses through the simple process of writing them down. Whether it be anger, loneliness, or fear, each can be tolerated, understood or sometimes accepted as satisfying.

**03 Sep 67**  10 Sep 67… 17 Sep 67… 24 Sep 67… 1 Oct 67… 8 Oct 67…
15 Oct 67—XXXXXX!

**19 Oct 67**  is getting close—Mag leaves 25 Sep, Tammy 26 Sep,
Pat 30 Sep and Mac 19 Oct with me. They all have their orders: Ft
Ord, Letterman and Fitzsimmons. The year is nearly over. No great
adventure, no heroic trials. I question the depth of my motivation for
volunteering. If nothing else, perhaps this Log will one day reveal
much about the drudgery of a situation such as this. As Steinbeck
remarks in *Travels with Charlie*: "Journeys choose their own time for
ending" (and tours of duty must do likewise). Vietnam is over for me.

**08 Sep 67**  Still no orders for Mac and me. The slides from Hong Kong
and Saigon have apparently been lost. Mail trickles in, most obviously
not from those avidly avowed correspondents of a year ago.

**10 Sep 67** Why is there so little to say on the eve of so many momentous
events?

**12 Sep 67** When I am lonely, I make things or write things down. Tonight
is such a time. Probably one month from now, Mac and I will board an
aircraft for the United States. Presently the turntable is transporting an
LP in circles at precisely (so it sounds) 33 & 1/3 revolutions per minute,
and it's mildly bizarre to reflect on the day's events.

We were moderately busy, a refreshing state of affairs.
Unexpectedly, Dian spiked a temp. He was ill for a brief period last
week, but with chloro and a sedative, there was much improvement.
We drew a blood culture, CBC and started D5&W with  He was
impassive. He responded to my gestures with a slight nod. He didn't
flinch. After an hour of sponging, the temp was down to 102.

This afternoon, three of the psychiatry patients restrained an MP
from attempting to kill a patient he had been assigned to guard. A call
to his CO for a replacement resulted in the CO demanding that we
release the patient for a "few days in the hotbox." The hotbox is a
conex box. In it, there is no light nor fresh air, and it is locked. It is a

steel box approximately 8' x 8' x 8' used for transporting and storing supplies. Of course, the patient was not released. Medication is a much more appropriate means of controlling an individual as destructive as he had been. As for the guard who felt provoked, perhaps he could have benefited from some medication also.

**19 Sep 67** Well, there was the vow that I would describe this experience, at least originally, and then the need to write it down—and then not any real feeling one way or another.

**20 Sep 67** We are in the midst of a war, and my spirit thinks only of its food, of escaping events we ultimately tolerated, for we could not choose otherwise. What had we thought it would be like here? When we saw films of sweat-drenched "troopers," was it only romantic? Did we not feel that sweat ourselves? When we read of poverty, was it with a disbelief of which even we were unaware? Did we think that people became diseased (with cholera, for example) from drinking chlorinated water?

The people—the people suffer; suffering is a feeling—they live. They are the war. The people live, and they die. They do not exist in some nebulous limbo with a sign at the entrance reading "Vietnamese Culture." They are real—they also sweat, they bleed, they stink from disease. Neither can they be classified in some Dewey-Decimal System. In this non-academic world, the people love, they lust, and when possible, they satisfy.

There is no movie set labeled "war zone—photographers welcome here." The war simply IS. It ebbs, it flows, it continues with or without documentation… most of all, it kills.

Did we see so little in those faces on TV last year? Did their voices mean so little to us? Were our tears of compassion, or of pity, only for our own synthetic lives? Was our desire to "serve" to help, an image of driving to and from a slum area, that we might "help" but not be touched? Well, we have been touched, and it doesn't feel anything like we thought it would.

I wished to learn about the "culture." I can tell you nothing of the VN religions. I can tell you nothing of VN eating habits, nor of the country's social taboos or national folk heroes, but I know how a Lambretta ride feels, what a thatched home looks like, and how the local market is arranged… I also jolly well know how a fighter jet sounds coming in a couple hundred feet overhead and that a rice paddy is not a place to dangle one's weary feet.

**25 Sep 67** Four nights from now, Pat, Mag, and Tam report to the 90th Replacement Center and, the next day, fly home. Apparently, it is as uncomplicated as that. Mac and I are next.

Next Tuesday (03 Oct) I appear before the RA (Regular Army) board. It's a bit reminiscent of attending grad school (with respect to the original decision to apply).

Sometime between 12 Oct and 19 Oct, Mac and I will leave for home. There is a "hail and farewell" this Friday evening.

One of the kids (medics) from Dustoff (helicopter rescue) was killed the other day. I didn't know him. The bullet went under his arm and across his chest…

Dian is better, having been placed on VSI (very seriously ill) but then SI, and he was finally removed from that status. His morale took a terrific tailspin for a while. We thought that he might not make it… but we were wrong…

Later: A long time ago, I saw a movie. Some conversation in the film disturbed me.

Scene: …an apartment, probably in NYC, though it doesn't matter... a discussion between a man and a woman; they are lovers; he is reviewing his daily session with his analyst when she responds to his mental groupings: "You speak as though you are a stranger to yourself. A person whose motivation you could only guess at."

I am learning. I have long been concerned with questions of motivation, especially with respect to one's values. The values of my friends are almost always different than the values of those with whom I work. How can this be? Do I pick my friends on that basis? Does their manner provide me with a certain pleasure that I dare not seek except vicariously? Am I also only capable of groping and guessing at my own motivation? It's somewhat like a game of social ping pong. Did I seek the military as a final territory where a pure motivation could exist? Perhaps this was one last attempt to justify the faith a child has or seeks. This purity is not present in either military or civilian life.

I overlooked the obvious when confronted with the disparity between the values of those with whom I work and those in rebellion. I think that for so many, in either instance, values are something to be mouthed without bringing one's actions into accord.

One is required by life to have tremendous courage. One must define one's own values, acknowledge those of others, perceive the deception of 99% of the adherents to same and emerge as one who can trust despite such knowledge. Only in this way, this refusal to abdicate one's convictions can one survive relatively intact. So many rebels must first have been the most moralistic of persons.

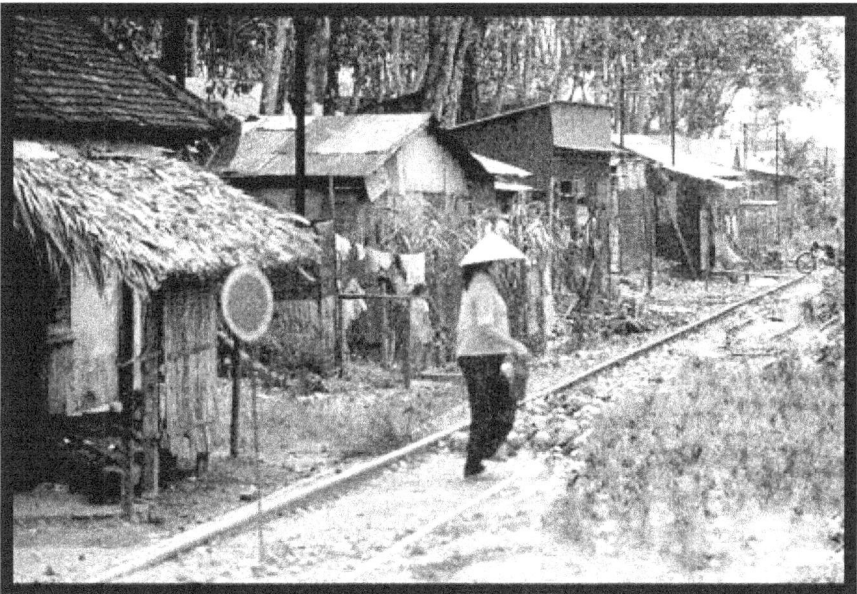

The Drudgery of Poverty

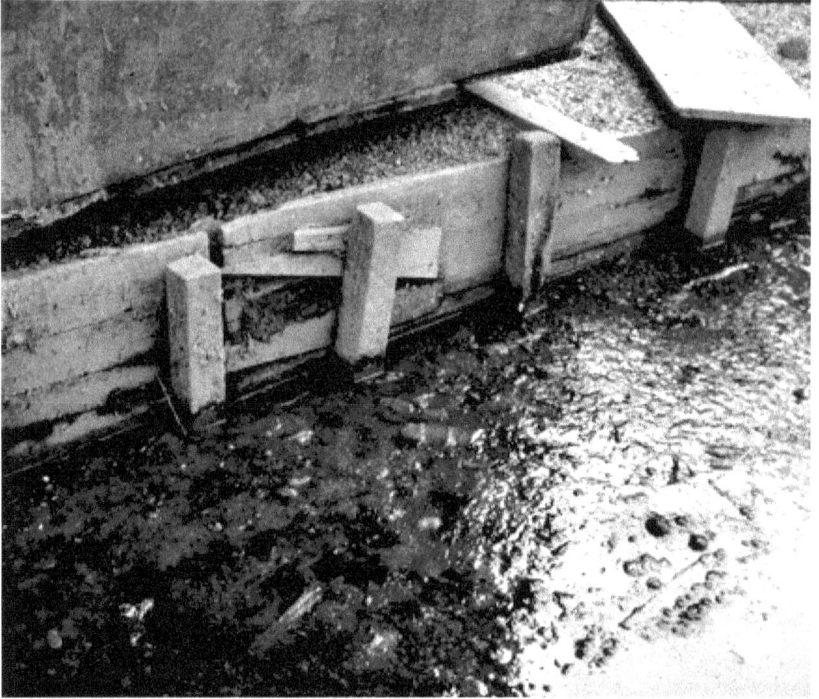

Water along the road in "town"

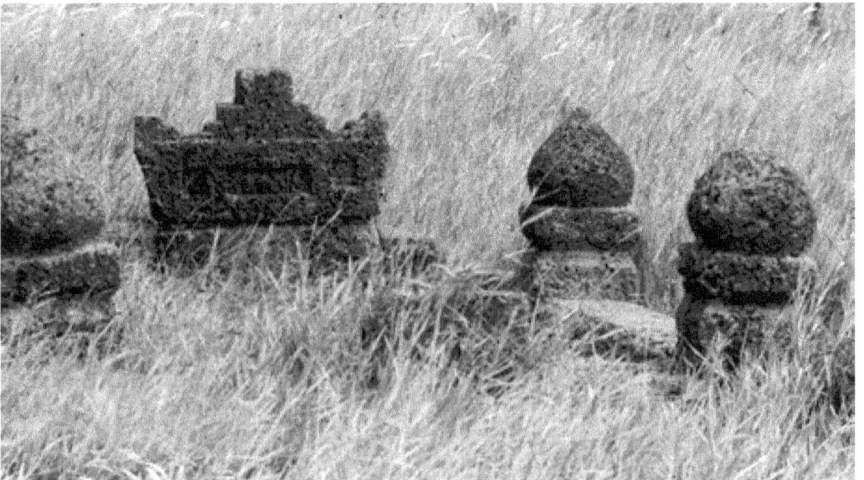

A Part of the Culture

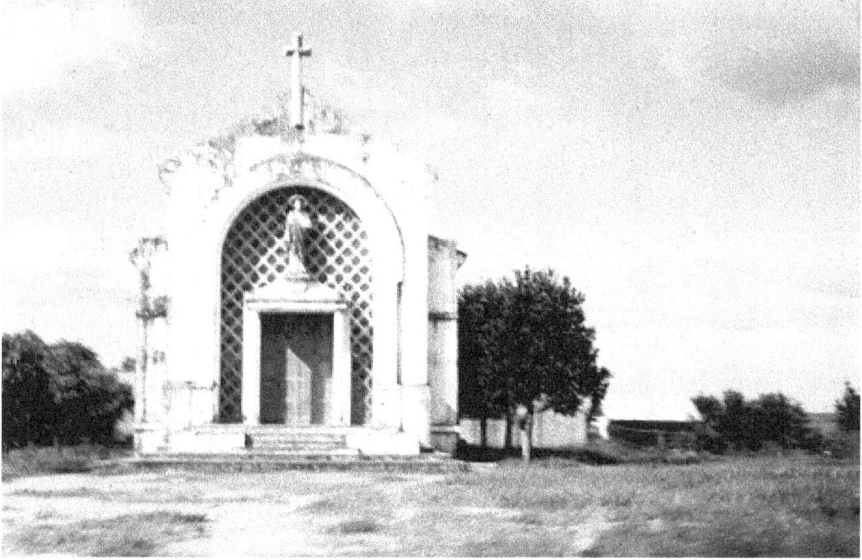

Another Aspect

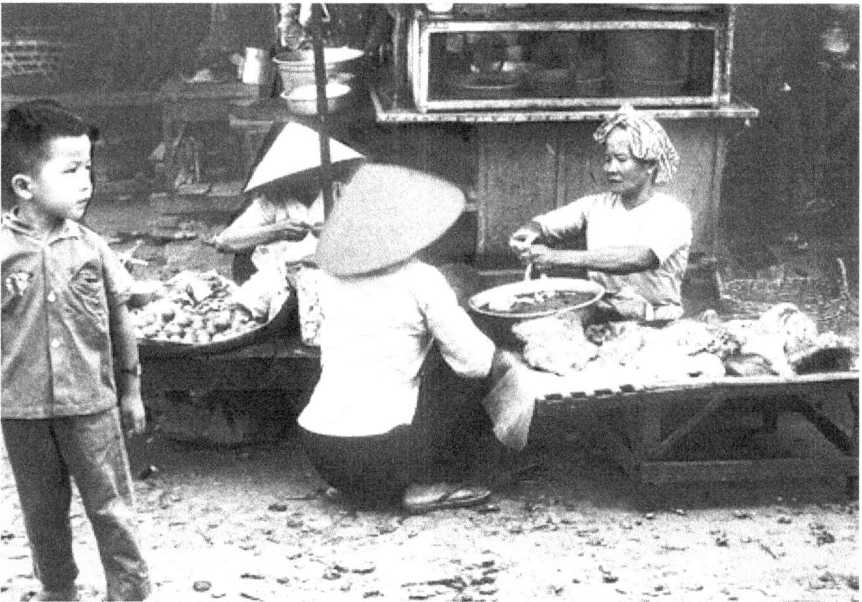

The Local Market

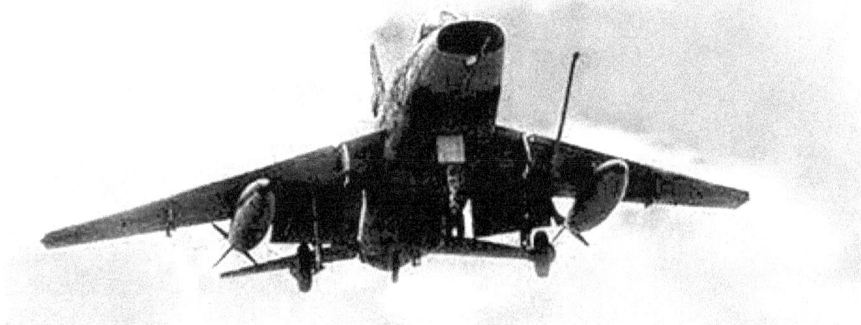

**At 200 Feet or 60 Feet Overhead?**

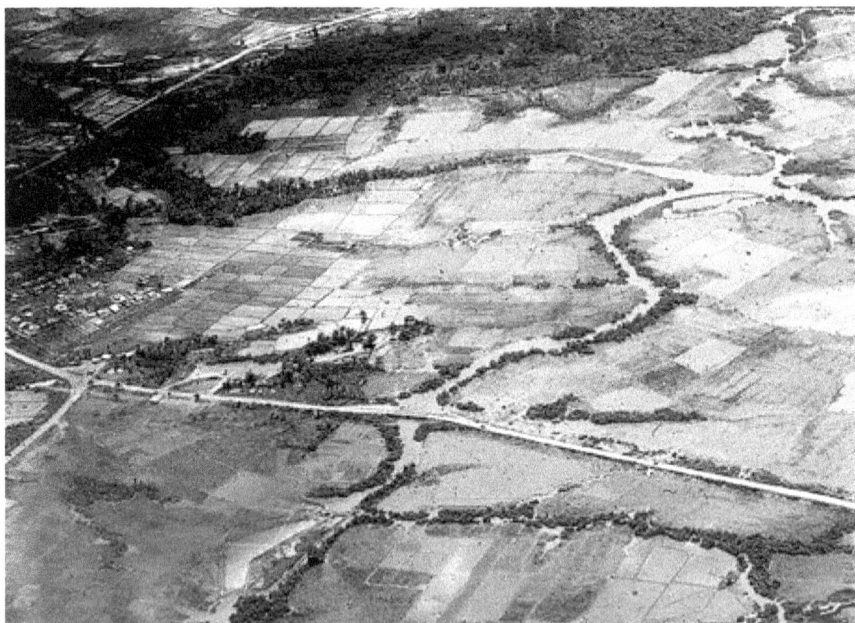

**Rice Paddies**

# Chapter 11: Going Home
# (06 Oct 67 – 27 Feb 69)

**06 Oct 67** I am 30 years old today. One week from tonight, we should leave RVN.

**13 Oct 67** The jukebox is playing: "Too many tears for one heart to be crying…"

There is no crying tonight, but neither is there an appreciable amount of laughter. Until people arrived to send us off, there was no laughter. There were mostly quiet conversations. We're going home. In one hour (0100), the bus leaves for Bien Hoa (the US Air Base is there).

**14 Oct 67** 0630 Yokota (Japan); we left Bien Hoa at 0115 Saturday, and it's still Saturday. Having flown away from RVN for R&R and leave, it didn't seem too different. I took a long last look when we flew over the only things discernable in the darkness... the ammo dump and the nearby hospital, the 93rd. While I slept until just before we landed in Japan, I had awakened earlier with a start, dreaming that we were crashing into a mountain. An uneasy thought of the length of the flight had crossed my mind, and I wondered if the men had any of these thoughts or if many were not wholly at peace in the safest environment they had known in the past year.

1100 In less than six hours, we should be home.

**Still 14 Oct 67** Twenty-four hours after leaving RVN: San Francisco The first day back in the US. How good it feels to have my hair washed and set. The beautician's fingers massage a certain anguish. I feel an impulse to thank her when she has but begun.

In the next chair, a middle-aged lady reviews "the terrible war" situation: "He's killing off at least 200 every day. I don't know why. Even the service men don't know why."

The beautician nods; uttering an emphatic agreement.

"You should see what they show these boys... fifty to sixty planes wiped out, bodies laying all around. My son's in the Air corps, so they show him, but they don't tell us half of what goes on."

"That's right. They don't dare."

"I think we need another Oswald."

I remain quiet. There's nothing to say to her, but I marvel at the statements.

**06 Dec 67** Thinking of it now, now that it is past, there is an uncertainty—a pride, yes, but an element of ill-defined pain. There are reactions that are not so easy to explain. There is an embarrassment when one is met with an exclamation of how "horrible it is." Is it? Was it? Was it for Me?... and one wants to explain that for me, there were sidewalks for transporting patients; there was a PX; and there was Armed Forces TV and radio; there was the club... but there was the other side as well, including having to convince someone who had been wounded, that when he was well he would have no choice but to return to the field.

It becomes apparent that such information makes others feel uncomfortable. Perhaps that's why they soon change the subject or just walk away. I am removed from them in these and in other ways. For example, I resent being told what I did or didn't "see"—a jet, a helicopter, a brightly lit night are private experiences for now they evoke private memories.

At times, I have had an impulse to reach out, to inflict pain—to make the harshness unavoidably apparent. For RVN was trust and friendship and excitement (when there was work to be done), and it was the temporarily inventoried gear of a dead man. It was being frightened and not having time to acknowledge such until the next day. It was gazing at a limb so mutilated that one wondered how it might be repaired—and, of course, too often, it wasn't. It was feeling guilty for having it soft. It was the endless waiting for time to pass. It was dirt and isolation.

**27 Feb 68** And Finally: It's been a long time. Today my thoughts overpowered my good sense. We've been at the Career Course (a 6-month middle-management focus) for 8 weeks. Last week I received approval of the RA (Regular Army) Commission. As I once noted, heaven only knows where that will lead.

I had discovered my current assignment upon reporting to BAMC (Brooke Army Medical Center, San Antonio, TX) in Nov. We study a great volume of material: the organization of the Army from DA (Department of Army) down to the deployment of each unit within the Divisions (offensive, defensive, and retrograde movements), automatic data processing, map reading and CBN (chemical, biological, and nuclear weapons).

Occasionally, there is vivid opportunity to recall Vietnam. This morning we saw a movie shot last spring at the 93rd. It moved about the buildings showing pre-op, OR, post-op, and one general view of sheets of rain splashing the ground into mud. I remember the day it was taken. There was no way of conceiving of today's possibility then. It's only real when you're there or when, such as today, you are unavoidably impressed with the gross impact of it all. For though I tried to compress it into one experience—one experience on film, it wasn't possible.

Tonight, while rummaging around, I came across a Christmas card—one received from one of our mama-sans last year. It was obviously secondhand. By some means, that lady had typed a holiday message on its back. In the stilted English of one feeling a need to relinquish use of her own tongue, she had wished me peace.

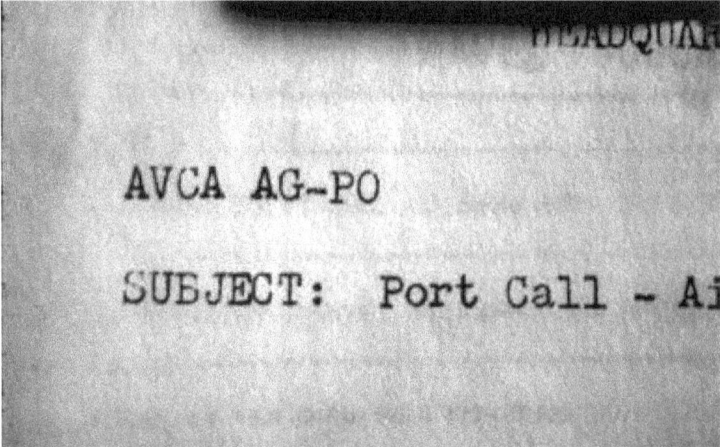

Orders for home

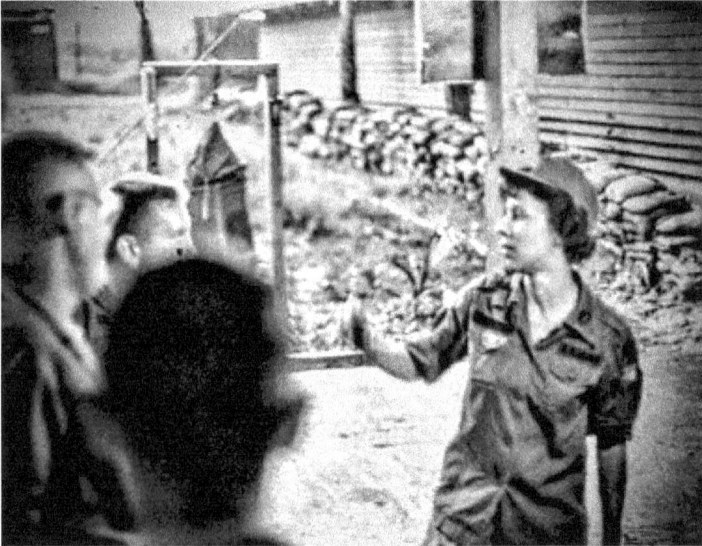

Saying goodbye

# A Part of What Daily Life Was

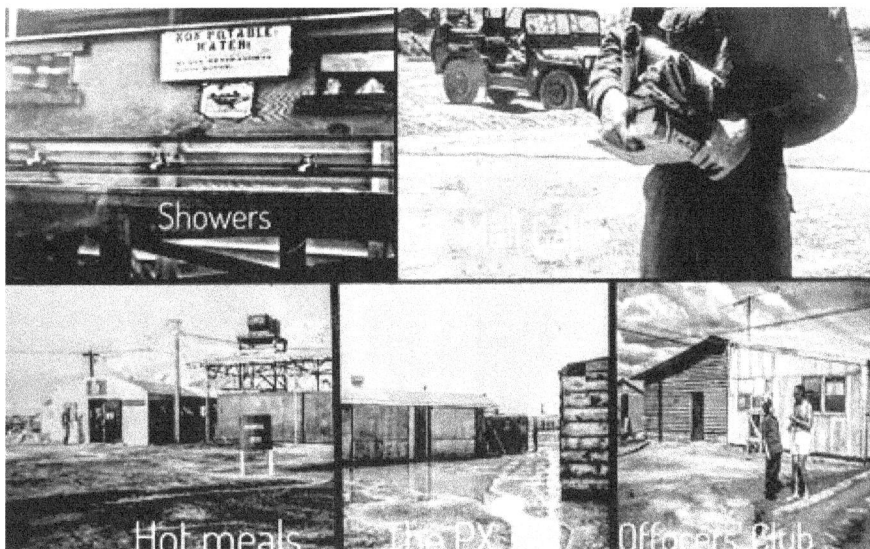

Fay Ferington

# *The Rest of It:*

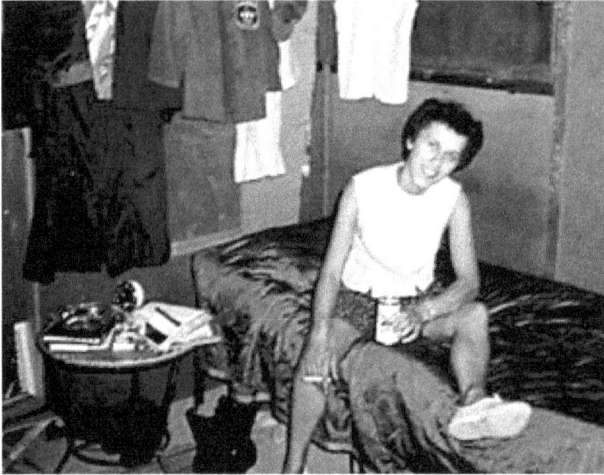

**Upon arrival in country**

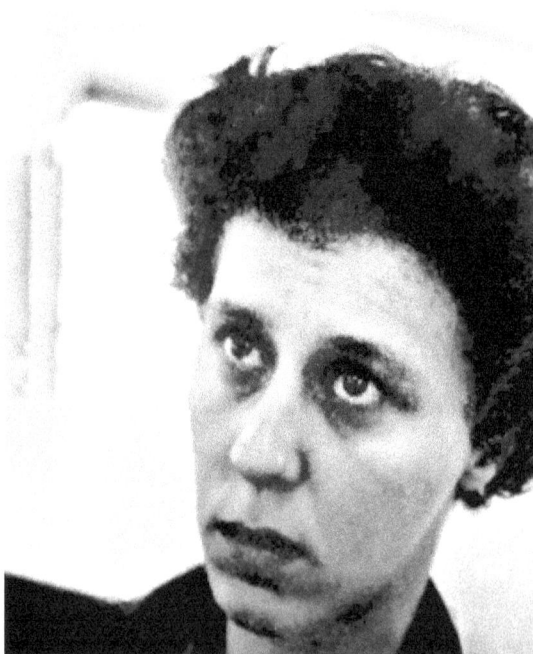

**Six months later**

# Appendix: Fragments

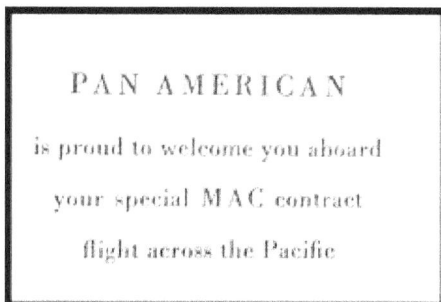

PAN AMERICAN

is proud to welcome you aboard

your special MAC contract

flight across the Pacific

**A special flight to a special place**

## Alert Plan

You will be concerned with two types of alerts at the 90th. They are red alerts and yellow alerts. In the event an alert should be called follow these instructions carefully and those given by battalion cadre personnel.

Yellow Alert - Notification will be three short blasts on the alert siren, or by announcement over the PA system. If an alert is called, go immediately to your assigned quarters and await further instructions.

Red Alert - Notification of a red alert will be incoming artillery, mortar rounds or one long blast on the post siren. Hit the ground immediately. If a drainage ditch is nearby, move quickly into it. If you are in the billets crawl under a bed and cover yourself with a mattress. If available, pull your duffle bag in close to you for added protection. Remain where you are until given the all clear signal. In the event of a ground attack (which is highly unlikely) remain indoors and stay out of the way of cadre personnel who are trained and equipped to react to the situation.

Termination of Alerts - The termination signal for either a yellow or red alert is one long blast on the siren.

**90th Replacement Center alert plan**

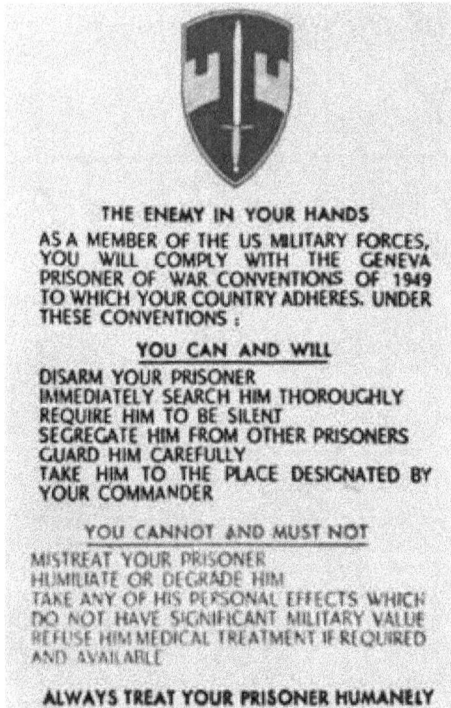

Geneva Convention (carried with ID)
Map of US Army hospitals in RVN

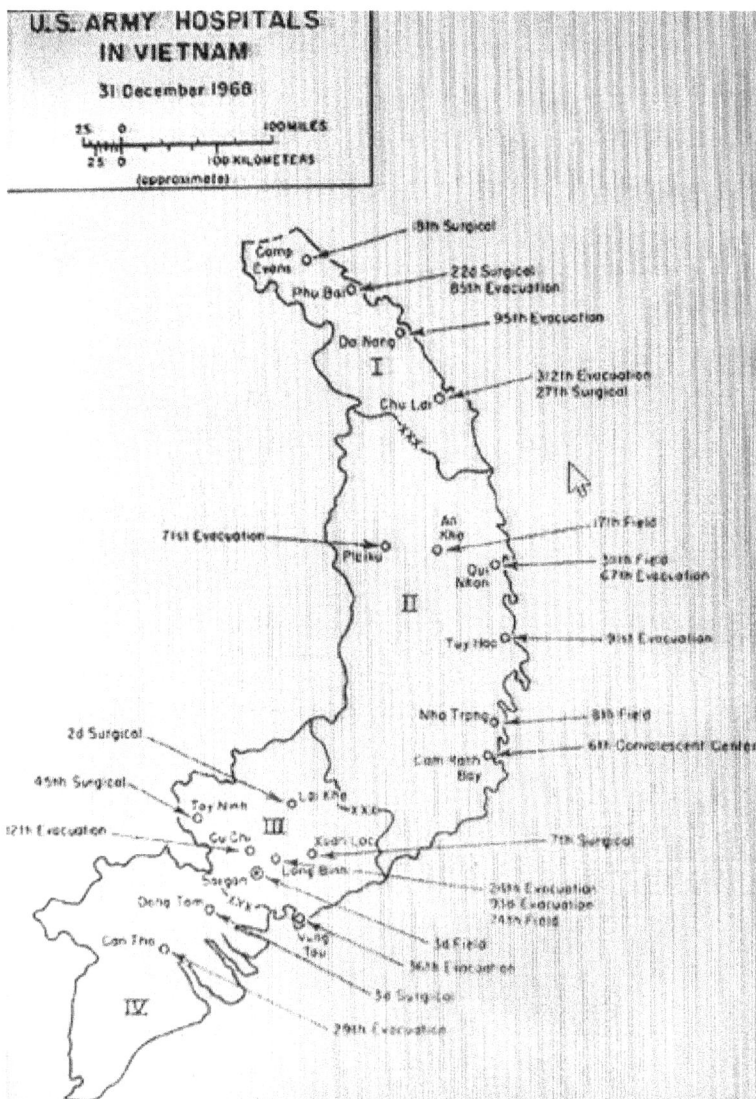

Map of US Army hospitals in RVN

# Land Control in RVN

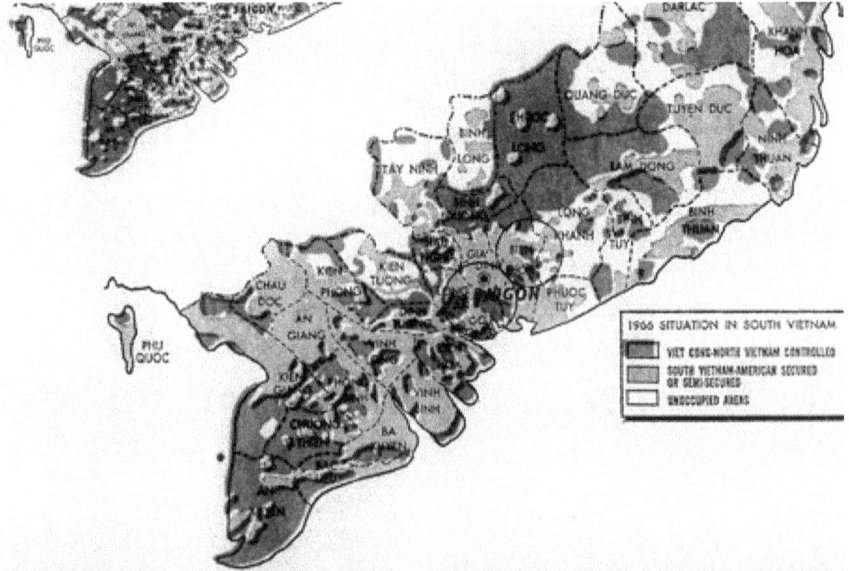

Map of 1966 land control in RVN
(large circle: Saigon; small circle: Bien Hoa)

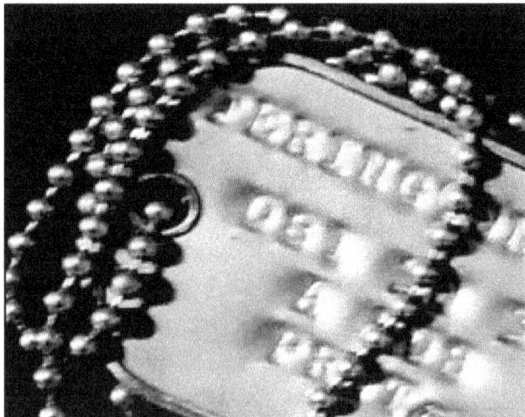

**Dog tags**

—They burned the flag of the greatest country in the world They slapped the face of 440,000 very young men who want nothing less than to be in Tay Ninh or Hill 861, but who get up + go every Time they're told to. They Turned their backs on the millions of people (many of them orphans, literally starving) we are trying to help to help Themselves.

**Letter to Warren**

# Operation Baby Lift

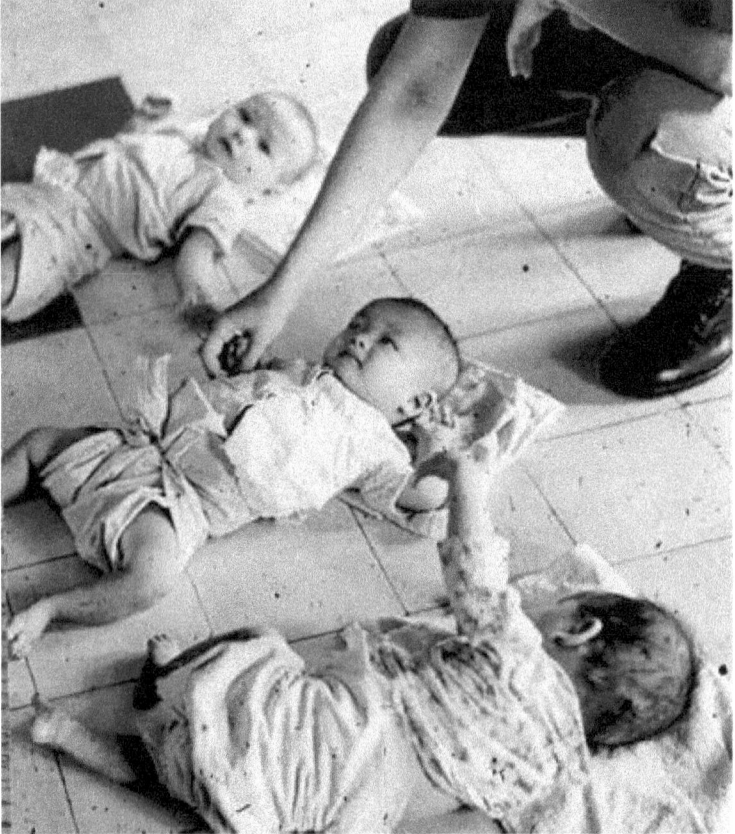

With the beginning of the fall of Saigon in April 1975, the military began to airlift Vietnamese orphans to Guam en route to the US. Over 2,500 were eventually placed with American families. Many were Amer-Asian.

Twelve minutes into the first flight, however, an explosion destroyed the plane's rear fuselage. It managed to return to Tan Son Nhut Airport, only to crash-land in a nearby rice paddy. Of the 328 people on board, there were 173 survivors. Of the 155 who died, there were 78 children and 77 adults.

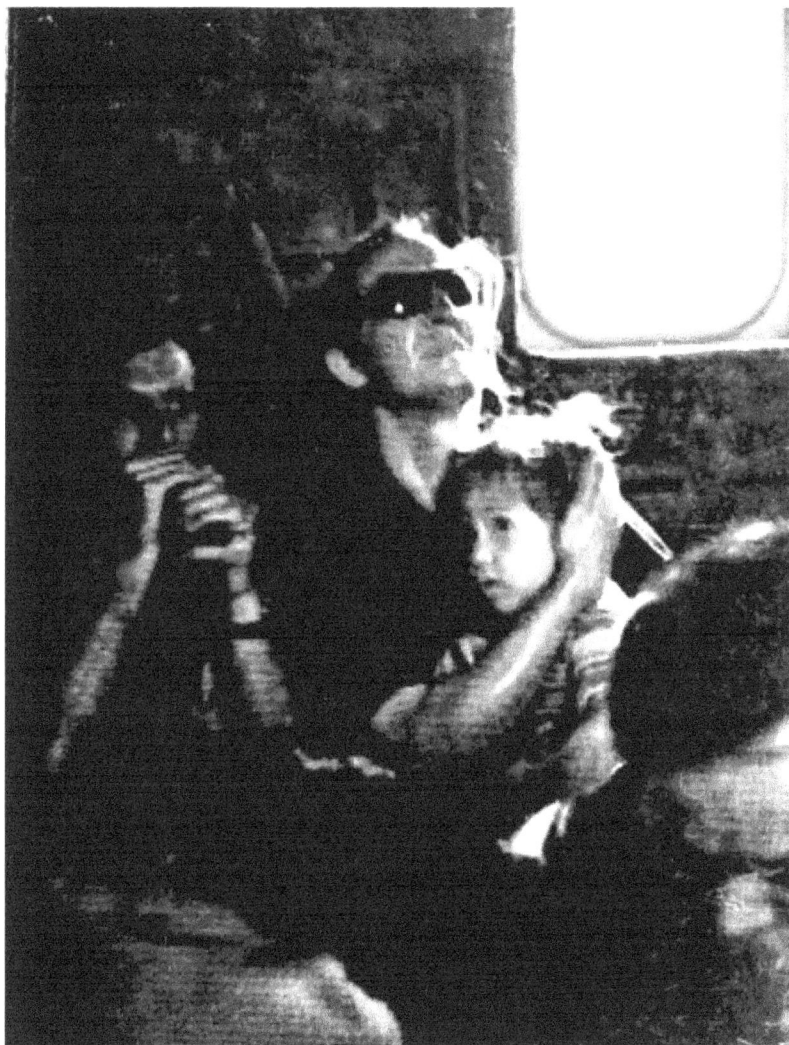

Inside one of the evacuation flights. It's not known if this was the flight that crashed.

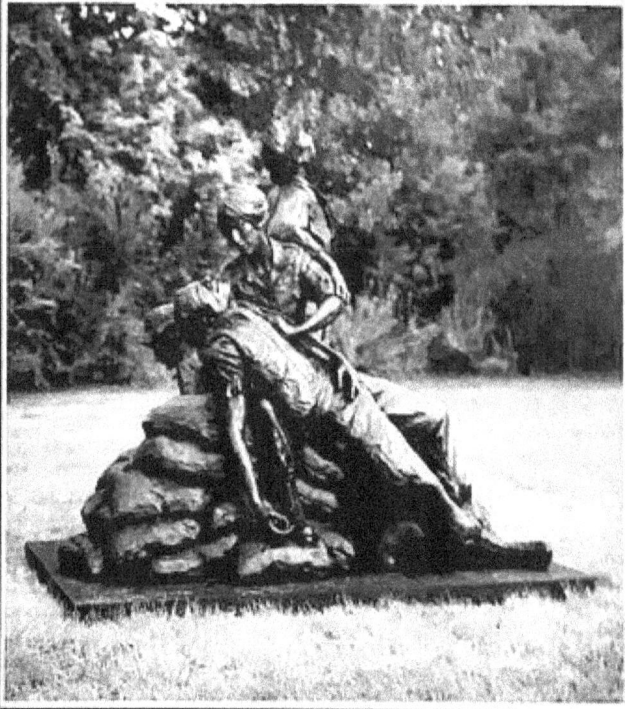

Women's Memorial

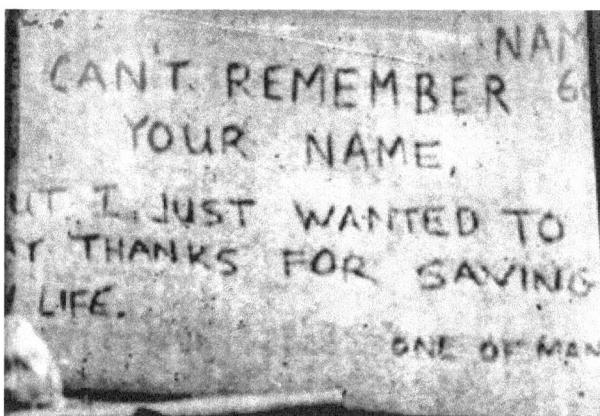

Note Left at Memorial

## General Colin L. Powell - July 29, 1993

...When this monument is finished, it will be for all time a testament to a group of American women who made an extraordinary sacrifice at an extraordinary time in our nation's history: the women who went to war in Vietnam...I knew you as nurses when you cared for those who were wounded and when you cared also, as one of them, for me.

...There are many scarred but living veterans who will never forget you nurses for helping to bring them back from the brink of eternity.

There are many others who are here only in spirit on the sacred Wall who will never forget you for trying so hard in those last desperate hours.

This monument will ensure that all of America will never forget that all of you were there, that you served, and that even in the depths of horror and cruelty there will always beat the heart of human love... and therefore our hope for humanity.

My fellow veterans - you and your sacrifice will never be forgotten. God Bless you all and thank you very much.

# Author's Note

I practiced nursing for forty years. My basic preparation was at SUNY, Buffalo graduating in 1960. I obtained a master's degree in psych-mental health in 1963. Most of my civilian and military career consisted of teaching and caring for patients in this practice area.

During eleven years of active duty, I served in Vietnam, provided mental health care for GIs returning from Vietnam and taught psych-mental health nursing at the Walter Reed Army Institute of Nursing. In my last assignment, I served in the personnel branch of the Army Surgeon General's Office, providing career development for junior nurse corps officers. I resigned from my regular army commission to pursue a PhD in nursing which I obtained in 1983. Throughout this effort and while appointed as a faculty member at the University of Wisconsin, I served in the reserve army nurse corps. I retired from the Army in 1991 and from civilian nursing in 1998.

Transforming the journal I kept in Vietnam into a published document was more complicated than I had anticipated, and I am deeply grateful to the following people for their assistance and encouragement:

Andy Millman and members of his writing class were the first persons to ever see the journal. Their reactions made me first think that it might contain a message. Members of my sister writing group, Joanne Storlie, Paula Sherman, and Mary Ellen Marcus, have been champions of my effort for several years.

Chris Chambers guided me in organizing the document into book form and writing a proposal.

My close friend Carol Berglund was there throughout this experience. She typed endlessly, assisted in determining the overall format of the book and was a meticulous researcher examining and crediting books written by other nurses who had served in Vietnam.

www.ingramcontent.com/pod-product-compliance
Lightning Source LLC
Chambersburg PA
CBHW031435270326
41930CB00007B/720